brain-centered treatment of addiction

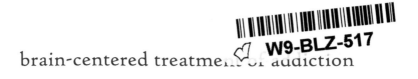

unchain your brain

10 steps to breaking the addictions that steal your life

Daniel G. Amen, M.D.

David E. Smith, M.D.

MindWorks Press
A Division of Amen Clinics, Inc.

MEDICAL DISCLAIMER

The information presented in this book is the result of years of practice experience and clinical research by the author. The information in this book, by necessity, is of a general nature and not a substitute for an evaluation or treatment by a competent medical specialist. If you believe you are in need of medical interventions please see a medical practitioner as soon as possible. The stories in this book are true. The names and circumstances of the stories have been changed to protect the anonymity of patients.

Published in the United States by MindWorks Press, a division of Amen Clinics, Inc., California. www.amenclinics.com

ISBN: 978-1-8865-5438-2

Printed in the United States of America

Cover design by Jaclyn Frattali

Also By Dr. Amen

Change Your Brain, Change Your Body, New York Times Bestseller

Change Your Brain, Change Your Body Cookbook

Magnificent Mind at Any Age, New York Times Bestseller

The Brain in Love

Making a Good Brain Great, Amazon Book of the Year

What I Learned from a Penguin: A Story on How to Help People Change

Preventing Alzheimer's

Healing Anxiety and Depression

New Skills for Frazzled Parents

Healing the Hardware of the Soul

Images of Human Behavior: A Brain SPECT Atlas

Healing ADD

How to Get out of Your Own Way

Change Your Brain, Change Your Life, New York Times Bestseller

ADD in Intimate Relationships

Would You Give 2 Minutes a Day for a Lifetime of Love

A Child's Guide to ADD

A Teenager's Guide to ADD

Mindcoach: Teaching Kids to Think Positive and Feel Good

Ten Steps to Building Values Within Children

The Secrets of Successful Students

Also By Dr. Smith

Drug Abuse Papers 1969. University of California, Berkeley, 1969. Editor

The New Social Drug: Cultural, Medical and Legal Perspectives on Marijuana. Prentice-Hall, Inc, 1970. Editor

Love Needs Care: A History of San Francisco's Haight Ashbury Free Medical Clinic. Little Brown & Co., 1971. Co-Author

The Free Clinic: Community Approaches to Health Care and Drug Abuse. STASH Press, 1972. Co-Editor

It's So Good, Don't Even Try It Once: Heroin in Perspective. Prentice-Hall, Inc., 1972. Co-Editor

Drugs in the Classroom. The C.V. Mosby Co., 1973. Co-Author

Uppers and Downers. Prentice-Hall, Inc., 1973. Co-Editor

Barbiturates: Their Use, Misuse and Abuse. Behavioral Publications, Inc., 1976. Co-Author

A Multicultural View of Drug Abuse: Proceedings of the National Drug Abuse Conference 1977. Schenkman and G.K. Hall Publishers, Cambridge, Massachusetts, 1978. Co-Editor

Amphetamine Use, Misuse and Abuse: Proceedings of the National Amphetamine Conference 1978. G.K. Hall Publishers, Boston, 1979. Co-Editor

Cocaine in America. Hazelden Foundation, Minneapolis, 1981, Smith DE, Wesson DR & Eiswirth NA.

PCP: Problems and Prevention. Kendall Hunt, Dubuque, Iowa, 1982. Co-Editor

The Little Black Pill Book. Bantam Books, New York, 1983. Medical Consultant

The Coke Book. Berkeley Books, New York, 1984. Medical Consultant

Cocaine: Helping Patients Avoid the End of the Line. 1985. Smith DE, Gold MS, Olden K & Dwyer BJ.

Treating the Cocaine Abuser. Hazelden Foundation, 1985. Smith DE & Wesson DR.

The Benzodiazepines: Current Standards for Medical Practice. MTP Press, Ltd., Boston, 1985. Co-Editor

The Physician's Guide to Psychoactive Drugs. The Haworth Press, New York, 1987. Seymour RB & Smith DE.

Guide to Psychoactive Drugs: An Up to the Minute Reference to Mind Altering Substances. Harrington Park Press, New York, 1987. Seymour RB & Smith DE.

Drugfree: A Unique, Positive Approach to Staying off Alcohol and Other Drugs. Facts on File Publications, New York, 1987. Seymour RB & Smith DE.

Still Free After All These Years: Two Decades With The Haight Ashbury Free Medical Clinic. Westwind Associates, Sausalito, 1987. Seymour RB & Smith DE.

Treating Cocaine Dependency. Hazelden Foundation, Minneapolis, 1988. Smith DE & Wesson DR.

Treating Opiate Dependency. Hazelden Foundation, Minneapolis, 1989. Wesson DR & Smith DE.

The New Drugs: Look Alike Drugs, Drugs of Deception and Designer Drugs. Hazelden Foundation, Center City, 1989. Seymour RB, Smith DE, Inaba DE & Landry MJ.

Crack and Ice: Treating Smokable Stimulant Abuse. Hazelden Foundation, Center City, 1992. Wesson DR, Smith DE, Steffens SC, Co-Editors.

Clinician's Guide to Substance Abuse. McGraw-Hill Medical Publishing Division, 2001. Smith, DE & Seymour, RB.

Dedication

For my patients, who are always my best teachers. —Daniel

To my wife Millicent, for introducing me to recovery. — David

TABLE OF CONTENTS

INTRODUCTION

David E. Smith, MD, and I are passionate about the work we do helping people break free from their addictions. The paths we took to arrive at this shared passion, however, couldn't be more different. David, who came from a long line of alcoholics, began his journey when he was sixteen years old. That's when his mother died and he had his first taste of alcohol. It was love at first drink. David had always been shy around women, but thanks to that drink, he felt a surge of confidence and vitality that buoyed his self-assurance around the opposite sex. Later that night, he threw up and blacked out. The next day, all he could think about was how alive he had felt while he was drinking and how he wanted to feel that way again—soon. The vomiting and blacking out part of the evening quickly faded from his thoughts.

David continued drinking and found that when he drank, he did some really stupid things he wasn't proud of. The next day, he would be filled with guilt about the things he had done, wondering "Why did I do that?" and promising himself he would never do it again. But then he would go out and have a drink, and it would trigger something in his brain that made him forget his good intentions, and he would get into trouble again. Eventually, he realized that alcohol was the problem, and he entered a 12-Step program. He had his last drink on January 1, 1966. David was finally sober, but he wasn't *"clean and sober."*

David simply switched from drinking alcohol to smoking marijuana and occasionally taking LSD. David loved the way the drugs made him feel spacey and even more important, he loved that he didn't do crazy things when he smoked pot. Psychedelic drugs were easy to find in the mid-1960s, especially in the Haight Ashbury district of San Francisco where David was living while going to the nearby UCSF School of Medicine. Haight Ashbury was the epicenter of the 1960s "turn on, tune in, drop out" counterculture and the place where rock legends like the Grateful Dead, Janis Joplin, Jimi Hendrix, The Doors, Jefferson Airplane, and concert promoter Bill Graham hung out.

While David was experimenting with mind-altering drugs, he was also using these same hallucinogens in research experiments on mice in the UCSF lab. He got his start in the addiction treatment field in 1965 when he began directing alcohol and drug screening at San Francisco General Hospital as part of his medical training. The following year, he started the renowned Haight Ashbury Free Medical Clinic, which catered to the music scene subculture by taking care of concertgoers who were having a bad LSD trip or who had overdosed. Eventually, they began helping the musicians as well. For example, when Janis Joplin OD'd on heroin, she was treated by the Clinics with narcan. The idea of "treating" drug problems was a revolutionary new concept at the time, and it would be years before anyone would consider treating the addiction rather than just the overdose.

For David, who had kicked his alcohol habit but had switched to smoking pot, it wasn't until the 1980s that he realized he needed to address his own addiction problem. He had finally come to the realization that even though smoking pot didn't make him do crazy things, it came with its own set of consequences. It compromised his ability to fully embrace a spiritual recovery program and it was creating a problem in his relationship with his significant other. He smoked his last joint in 1987, went into recovery, and has been clean and sober ever since. He has dedicated his professional career to helping others break the drug and alcohol addictions he faced.

I, on the other hand, didn't have any alcoholics in my family and was also sixteen years old the first time I got drunk. My introduction to alcohol involved guzzling half a bottle of champagne and a six-pack of Michelob. I spent the rest of the night acting like an idiot and throwing up in the bathroom of my brother's apartment. The next day, I could barely drag myself out of bed, and had to go to work at my father's grocery store.

On this particular day, my dad found out I was hung over. When you come from a family of seven children there are few secrets, so my dad thought it would be a good idea for me to work in the liquor department that day. Having to handle all those bottles of alcohol when I was already reeling from a hangover made me feel even worse. I felt so sick, it took me about three days to get back to normal.

In my memory, there wasn't anything fun about drinking. All I remembered about it was how sick it made me and how embarrassed I felt. Since then, I rarely touch alcohol, and I have never tried an illicit drug. But that doesn't mean I have never had any bad habits or that I am not vulnerable to addiction.

In my professional life as a psychiatrist, neuroscientist, and brain imaging specialist, I have realized that everybody is potentially at risk for addiction and that drugs and alcohol aren't the only kinds of addictions that can damage the brain and ruin your life. I have also discovered that our daily behaviors and habits can either hurt our brains and make us more vulnerable to addiction, or they can help our brains and protect us from addiction. For more than twenty years, I have been treating people with all sorts of addictions to help them change their behaviors, enhance their brain function, beat their addictions, and improve the quality of their lives.

Although David and I have both arrived at similar places in our careers, our connection goes beyond a purely professional collaboration. We first crossed paths more than fifteen years ago. One of David's family members was in crisis, and the family came to me when they were desperate for help. They had heard about my work with brain imaging, which was very controversial at the time, and hoped it might be beneficial in their case. The brain imaging did help, but it was the quality of our relationship that impressed David and his family. As David's family member improved, David and I—and our families—forged a deep and lasting friendship that straddles our professional and personal lives.

Our two stories show very clearly that all people and all brains are not the same. Most people can drink or experiment with drugs without becoming addicted. For some people, however, a single gulp of alcohol or hit from a crack pipe can lead to a lifetime battle with addiction. For others, drugs and alcohol aren't a problem, but they can't break their addiction to gambling, video games, Internet pornography, shopping, sex, food, smoking, social networking, texting, or working. What is it about our brains that make some of us more vulnerable to addiction than others? And what can we do to break free from these addictions? These are some of the questions we have heard from thousands of patients who inspired us to write this book together.

This book is divided into two parts. The first part helps you understand addiction and why some of us get sucked into its grasp. We will use the latest brain imaging research to show you what goes on inside the brain that makes some people more likely to fall into and stay in the grips of addiction. You'll learn to identify some of the signs of addiction in yourself or in those you care about, whether it's your spouse, your child, your grandchild, your parent, your friend, your roommate, your student, your coworker, or your boss. This part will also shed light on common daily behaviors that might be setting you (or a loved one) up for addictions.

The second part of this book focuses on breaking the chains of addiction so you can take control of your life instead of letting your addiction control you. The steps to unchain your brain are simple but not necessarily easy. After working with thousands of people with addictions, we know just how tough it can be to overcome addiction. But we have seen it work over and over again and know that it is one of the most rewarding things you can ever do in life. Breaking an addiction will improve every aspect of your life, including your family life, your relationships, your career, and your school life. In this part, you will find prescriptions for daily life that will help you remain free from your addictions so you can be happier, healthier, and more successful in everything you do.

To help you break the addictions that steal your life, this part will include a wealth of tips and strategies, including the following:

➤ One decision that will change your life—making the decision to unchain your brain.

➤ Four areas of your life you need to address to prevent relapse.

➤ Five natural supplements that can soothe your brain and reduce your cravings.

➤ Seven steps parents can take now to prevent addictions in children.

➤ Ten daily behaviors that will enhance brain function and help you beat your addictions.

➤ Fifteen strategies for dealing with the people who try to sabotage your recovery.

David often says that addiction is like getting on an elevator that only goes in one direction: down. You get on at the first floor, and as your addiction progresses, you keep going down, down, down to the second floor, third floor, fourth floor and so on until you hit the bottom at about the twelfth floor. You can get off the elevator at any time, and the earlier you get off, the easier it is to reclaim control of your life. It is our goal that this book will inspire you to get off that elevator before you end up at the bottom.

How Addictions Steal Your Life

When you are chained by an addiction, it affects every area of your life. Addiction ruins lives, devastates families, destroys relationships, negatively impacts your career, decreases your ability to perform well in school, and causes health problems. People with addictions are more likely to get divorced, less likely to graduate from high school or college, less likely to get promoted at work, and more likely to develop diseases related to their addiction. Addiction also affects our society as a whole and burdens us all. Here are some alarming statistics about the dangerous effects of addiction.

> It is estimated that there were nearly one million drug-related deaths annually in the U.S. from 2004 to 2008.

> Smoking is the number-one preventable cause of death.

> Being overweight or obese ranks third on the list of preventable causes of death.

> Obesity, often caused by an addiction to unhealthy food, costs our society over $145 billion annually.

> Medical costs for an obese person are 42 percent higher than those of a healthy-weight person.

> Morbid obesity is associated with more than thirty medical conditions and diseases, including an increased risk for Alzheimer's disease, diabetes, and stroke.

> Alcohol abuse is the seventh most common preventable cause of death.

> We spend close to $500 billion alone on morphine addiction when you factor in healthcare costs, crime and criminal justice costs, accidents, and lost employment.

> It is estimated that the cost of drug abuse has grown to approximately $1 trillion annually in America.

Addiction is far more prevalent than you might imagine, and it can affect anyone—you, your spouse, your child, your best friend, your neighbor, your teacher, your coworker, your plumber, even your doctor. Just take a look at the latest numbers.

> More than 23 million Americans age twelve and older are affected by substance abuse or dependence—that's nearly one in ten Americans.

- One in five Americans between the ages of sixteen and fifty-nine admits to using drugs.

- Nearly one in ten adolescents between the ages of twelve and seventeen surveyed said they had used illicit drugs within the past month.

- One in five drinkers reported drinking five or more drinks on at least one day in the past year.

- More than 28 percent of youths aged twelve to twenty reported drinking in the past month. In some states, the number jumped as high as 40 percent.

- Among underage drinkers, 19 percent identified themselves as binge drinkers and about 6 percent considered themselves to be heavy drinkers. Among young adults aged eighteen to twenty-five, more than 42 percent reported binge drinking, and nearly 16 percent reported heavy drinking.

- Approximately two million adults meet the criteria for pathological gambling. Another four to six million have serious problems with gambling.

- One in ten people who play video games shows signs of addictive behavior.

- Ten percent of adults admit to being addicted to Internet pornography.

- Between 2 and 8 percent of Americans have a compulsive shopping addiction.

- In the U.S., more than 47 million people are smokers.

- In the U.S., two-thirds of people are overweight and one-third are obese.

➤ About 62 percent of high-earning individuals in the U.S. work more than fifty hours a week, which is the criteria for addiction to work, 35 percent work more than sixty hours, and 10 percent work more than eighty hours.

THE PROBLEM
Most people with addiction problems do not think the brain has anything to do with their addiction

Why is addiction so pervasive, and what can we do to prevent and treat it? Many government, community, school, and parent organizations as well as thousands of treatment specialists and recovery centers are desperately trying to pinpoint the answer. In all of the fact-finding and hand-wringing, we are missing the essential organ of intervention: the brain. The brain is the supercomputer that runs your life. It plays a central role in your vulnerability to addiction and your ability to recover and maintain sobriety. Understanding the brain's role in addiction, prevention, and treatment is the key to helping people break free from your addictions. Once addiction specialists, recovery centers, and people with addictions recognize the importance of the brain, they will be better able to treat the problem so you can enhance the quality of your life.

Until then, people will continue to fuel their addictions with daily habits and actions that pollute the brain and make it even harder for them to break free from those addictions. Working at ever-frenzied paces, not getting enough sleep, and living with strained relationships stresses the brain and lowers brain function, which makes it harder to fight addiction. Eating fast food diets, guzzling caffeinated drinks, and gobbling sugary snacks deprives the brain of proper nutrients, decreasing your ability to think clearly and make good decisions. Isolating yourself from friends and family in order to hide your addiction also has a negative affect on your brain that can intensify addictive behaviors.

Brain dysfunction is the number-one reason why people fall victim to addiction, why they can't break the chains of addiction, and why they relapse.

THE PROMISE

By taking the necessary steps to unchain your brain and improve brain function, you will be able to break the addictions that steal your life

Once you make the decision to unchain your brain, you can learn how to keep your brain healthy and stay away from addiction. *Unchain Your Brain* is a practical, easy-to-read, step-by-step guide that introduces you to the most up-to-date neuroscience research on how to optimize brain function as well as the latest trends in treatment and recovery so you will have a better chance of living an addiction-free life. Improving brain function increases your ability to think clearly, make good decisions, love, work, and learn. This book is also based on decades of personal experience treating patients with addiction and seeing first-hand what helps them kick the addiction habit.

In his forty-five-year career in the field of addiction medicine, David E. Smith has served as the president of the American

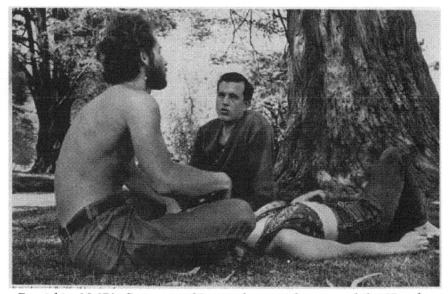

David in 1967's Summer of Love, the year he started the Haight Ashbury Free Medical Clinic

18

Society of Addiction Medicine and the California State Department of Alcohol and Drug Programs and is currently the medical director of Center Point, a therapeutic community focused on those coming out of the criminal justice system, and the chair of adolescent addiction treatment at Newport Academy, a gender-specific residential treatment center for teens with substance abuse and co-occurring disorders. In his vast experience, he has successfully treated thousands of patients addicted to drugs and alcohol. In this book, he will be sharing many of the insights he has learned to help you with your own recovery.

I am the CEO and medical director of the Amen Clinics, which has amassed the world's largest database of brain scans—more than 57,000 scans—related to behavior, including addiction. For more than twenty years, I have been looking at the brain on a daily basis using a sophisticated study called brain SPECT imaging. I have looked at healthy brains and tens of thousands of brains in trouble. I have looked at the brains of young children, teenagers, adults, and the elderly. I have looked at brains on drugs, on alcohol, on prescription medications, on supplements, on prayer and meditation, on gratitude, and on a wide variety of psychological and biological treatments. I have used brain imaging to help our patients win the battle against their addictions to food, gambling, sex, video games, shopping, pornography, and more. At the Amen Clinics, the goal is to look at, optimize, and restore the brain. This book will contain many of the lessons we have learned in the process.

THE PROGRAM

Our program contains the ten steps you need to know to have the best brain possible to help you fight the addictions that steal your life. It starts with the basic principles of brain science as they apply to addiction and recovery. It reveals how addictions get started and how they get stuck in your brain. It explores how each individual's brain and addiction is unique and how a one-size-fits-all treatment method will never work for every addict. It alerts you to the daily habits that might be making you or your loved ones more vulnerable to addiction. It shows you how addiction may be a symptom of other underlying brain dysfunctions and how treating those problems can be a big part of the answer to overcoming addiction.

This practical program also gives you ten steps to optimize brain function so you can break free from your addictions and avoid relapse. It teaches you to protect your brain from injuries, a lack of sleep, and toxic substances—such as too much caffeine, sugar, or nicotine—which have been shown to trigger relapses in some people. It emphasizes the need to develop a positive social network to enhance brain function and help you maintain sobriety. It gives practical instructions on what and when to eat so your brain is properly nourished to improve your ability to think clearly and make better decisions. A critical component of the program is physical exercise, which boosts blood flow and other positive nutrients to the brain and has been shown to reduce cravings in recovering addicts. The program shows you how to rid your brain of bad thoughts (ANTs—automatic negative thoughts) that interfere with good judgment, love, and health.

Ways to counteract stress are a very important part of the program, as stress is a common cause for relapse and because chronic stress disrupts neural pathways and kills cells in the memory centers of the brain. Another important part of the program deals with natural supplements that can help your brain and your sobriety. Finally, the program offers simple steps parents can take now that will help prevent their children from falling into the stranglehold of addiction. All of my children are vulnerable to addictions from their genetic history on their mother's side. This is an issue I have thought about for a very long time.

Part One

UNDERSTANDING THE CHAINS OF ADDICTIONS

Chapter 1

WHO ME?

How Do You Know if You, or Someone You Love, Has a Problem
Know the warning signs of addiction.

You know you have a problem when:

- Your cat's gone without food for three days.

- Your wife, who used to adore you, is always mad at you … and it isn't just during the PMS period.

- Your favorite phrase is, "What did I do last night?"

- Your rent check is stuck inside an overdue library book that you left … somewhere.

- Your favorite band is playing in town, but you would rather spend the night alone with your _____ (insert your bad habit of choice here).

The first step to unchaining your brain is to admit when you have a problem. Recognizing that you have a problem isn't easy. For many people, addiction creeps up slowly and the changes are hard to notice. By the time you are in the grips of addiction, your brain has effectively been rewired and it drives you to continue your bad behavior in spite of the negative consequences. A little objectivity can help you determine if your bad habits have become a real problem and can help you detect addiction in your child, spouse, parent, friend, coworker, or sibling.

Take this quick quiz to find out if you might have a problem.

This questionnaire is called the CAGE Assessment and it has been used for decades in the addiction field to help identify problem drinking. These same questions can also help you pinpoint problems with other substances and behaviors. Simply substitute the word "drinking" with "smoking," "prescription drug use," "overeating," "Internet porn viewing," "shopping," "gambling," or whatever your bad habit may be.

CAGE Assessment

Have you ever felt you should **C**ut down on your drinking ... or other behavior?

- o Yes
- o No

Have people **A**nnoyed you by criticizing your drinking ... or other behavior?

- o Yes
- o No

Have you ever felt bad or **G**uilty about your drinking ... or other behavior?

- o Yes
- o No

Have you ever had a drink ... or engaged in other behavior ... first thing in the morning (as an "**E**ye opener") to steady your nerves or get rid of a hangover?

- o Yes
- o No

If you answered "yes" to two or more of these questions, then you may have a problem.

Continued Use Despite Consequences

Another definition of addiction that David and I like has to do with continued use despite consequences. Ask yourself the following question.

Do you drink, overeat, or engage in other addictive behaviors despite significant negative consequences of the behavior in your health, your relationships, your money, or with the law?

O Yes
O No

If you answered yes, then it is time to take a hard look at it.

Signs and Symptoms of Addiction

Addiction impacts every aspect of your life, including your physical health, mental and emotional health, social life, and core values. The signs and symptoms of addiction can be biological, psychological, social, or spiritual, and most people with a problem will exhibit signs in several if not all of these areas. These areas are called the four pillars of addiction and healing, and you will learn much more about them in upcoming chapters. Here are some real-life examples to help you determine if you or someone you love has an addiction.

Five-foot-five-inch Keisha weighed 145 pounds when she went away to college. With all the desserts on display in the cafeteria, she couldn't help herself from taking one of each. She gained about twenty pounds while in college and continued to gain another ten pounds every year. When she got engaged, she tried to give up sweets so she could lose weight for her wedding, but she couldn't resist the cravings and never lost the weight.

After she got married, she didn't want her husband to know about her dessert habit so she started hiding candy bars, cookies, and brownies in her desk at work, in her underwear drawer at home, and in the glove compartment of her car. She would lie to him and say that she was following a healthy diet to try to lose weight and claimed the diet just wasn't working for her. When she ballooned to 245 pounds and was diagnosed with type 2 diabetes, Keisha continued to devour several candy bars and at least one box of triple fudge cookies a day.

Is Keisha addicted to overeating? You bet.

Cole was a shy, quiet sixteen-year-old who loved playing the piano and being on the math club. When one of his older brother's friends introduced him to cocaine, he immediately loved the way it melted away his shyness and made him feel more outgoing, talkative, and energetic. When he used it, his friends said he was the life of the party, and girls seemed to like him more. So he started using it whenever he went to a party. Then he began snorting a few lines before school events, and then he did it every morning before he got to school. He rarely felt hungry anymore and lost about fifteen pounds, leaving him rail thin.

When Cole was high, he talked a mile a minute and fidgeted in his seat in class. But when the effects wore off, he went back to his old introverted self, felt depressed, and could barely muster the energy to get off the couch. He quit taking piano lessons, dropped out of the math club, and dumped all his old friends in order to spend more time with his new drug buddies. When he couldn't get his hands on any cocaine, he couldn't stop thinking about it and lashed out at his parents and younger sister whenever they asked him if he was using drugs.

Is Cole addicted to cocaine? Absolutely.

Garrett, thirty-six, worked as a sales executive and was expected to wine and dine his clients. On business trips, he would take clients to trendy bars and restaurants. On a typical night, he would have a few beers before dinner, then a couple glasses of wine with dinner, then several more beers after dinner. By the end of the night, he was usually pretty wasted. Even though Garrett was married and loved his wife, whenever he got drunk, he got the urge to hook up and would end up inviting some waitress or bartender to go back to his hotel and have sex. As soon as the woman would leave, Garrett would feel terribly guilty about cheating on his wife and would promise to himself that he would never do it again. But he couldn't stop.

Eventually, he started spending extra days on business trips so he could indulge in his drinking and "sexcapades." When his wife would ask him why he was doing so much more traveling, he lied and said his new boss was forcing him to spend more time on the road. At home, Garrett's wife would monitor his drinking and try to limit him to just a couple drinks a night, which would infuriate him. When she mentioned that she was worried he might have a drinking problem, he would fly off the handle. He soon found that whenever he was home, he couldn't stop thinking about getting back out on the road.

Does Garrett have a drinking problem? Definitely. Is he a sex addict? It's possible, however, he has never had extramarital sex when he wasn't drunk, so the hypersexuality may actually be a symptom of his drinking problem.

Shelley, forty-five, had been suffering from back pain for years. She'd visited chiropractors, physical therapists, neurologists, and spine surgeons. None of the exercises, stretches, or other therapies seemed to help. Eventually she opted for surgery and was given a prescription for the painkiller OxyContin for post-surgical pain. Finally, she felt some relief from the chronic agony. She wasn't sure if it was the surgery or the painkiller that was helping her so when the prescription ran out, she asked for a refill... just in case.

When that supply ran low, she felt the pain returning and got a higher dosage. The next time she asked her physician for a refill, he refused. This really ticked her off, and Shelley complained to her friends that her doctor was a jerk. She went to another doctor and got a new prescription, then saw another physician for an additional supply. When these doctors cut her off, Shelley felt terrible, called in sick from work for a whole week, and didn't even get out of bed to take a shower the entire time.

She started telling her friends that her doctor had just transferred to a new hospital and wasn't in their system yet so he couldn't write any new prescriptions for now, so could they possibly give her any pain pills they might have at home just until her doctor got his prescribing privileges back? Then she found out about a doctor who supposedly would give her a new supply without too many questions, and she drove two and a half hours to see him.

Is Shelley addicted to painkillers? No doubt about it.

While these examples may seem pretty clear cut, many times, it is difficult to know if you just have a bad habit or if it is really an addiction. To help you make a determination, take a look at some of the many warning signs of addiction below and see if you recognize yourself or a loved one in any of them.

Biological Signs and Symptoms

Biological signs include changes to physical health and appearance and include, but are not limited to, the following.

- Sudden increases or decreases in activity level or energy level
- Weight loss or weight gain
- A lack of personal hygiene
- Strange body odor
- Changes in the health of skin and teeth
- Red, watery, glassy eyes or a runny nose that is not due to cold or allergies
- Changes in eating habits
- Changes in sleeping patterns
- Feeling sick or hung over
- Blacking out or forgetting what happened while under the influence
- Using increasing amounts of a substance

- Developing diseases and conditions related to your bad habit
- Inability to quit without experiencing cravings or withdrawal

Psychological Signs and Symptoms

Addiction takes a real toll on emotional health and can result in many psychological symptoms. Here are some of the many signs and symptoms associated with problem behavior.

- Mood swings
- Feelings of depression
- Irritability
- Anger
- Negative attitude
- Inability to focus
- Lack of motivation
- Loss of interest in favorite activities
- Denying or minimizing the consequences of using the substance or engaging in the behavior
- Defensiveness—getting annoyed or irritated whenever someone questions you about your habits
- Feelings of guilt about your bad habits
- Feeling anxious, depressed, or irritable when you are unable to engage in the behavior or use the substance
- Using the substance or doing the behavior in response to feelings of sadness or to alleviate stress
- Spending your day thinking about when you will have your next chance to use the substance or do the behavior
- Feeling powerless to change your behavior

Social Signs and Symptoms

Changes in a person's social life are common when addiction kicks in. Some of the changes to look for are listed here.

- Negative changes in work performance—calling in sick,

showing up late, missing meetings, trouble meeting deadlines, problems with coworkers

- Negative changes in school performance—skipping classes, being tardy, falling grades, problems with classmates and teachers
- Withdrawal from family and friends
- Neglecting responsibilities—not taking care of children or pets, foregoing household chores, not finishing homework, forgetting to pay the bills
- Shifting away from former friends and becoming friends with people who share the same addiction
- Becoming antisocial
- For teens and children, hanging out with older kids
- Spending more and more time engaging in the behavior
- Avoiding situations where you can't engage in the behavior
- Your life has become unmanageable

Spiritual Signs and Symptoms

In this context, "spiritual" doesn't mean "religious." It refers to your core values and morals, which are typically compromised in people with addictions. For example, before you became a slave to your habit, you probably never would have lied to your spouse, stolen money from a friend, or forgotten to pick up the kids from school. When you become entangled in addiction, however, you start to do things you used to think were wrong. The following are signs of a broken moral compass.

- Breaking rules at home, at school, or in the community
- Keeping secrets
- Cheating
- Lying to family, friends, significant others, coworkers, and others
- Stealing to fuel your habit
- Hiding things
- Selling personal items to get extra cash to fund your habit
- Breaking promises and making excuses
- Using street language, drug language, or jargon only people

with your habit would understand

As you look at these lists of signs and symptoms, be honest with yourself about the changes in your behavior and life. Take a pen and circle the signs and symptoms that sound like you or a loved one. The more symptoms you circle, the more likely it is that there is a problem. Unless you recognize and admit that you have a problem, you will not be able to unchain your brain.

UNCHAIN YOUR BRAIN CHECKLIST

- ✓ Take the CAGE Assessment to see if your behavior or substance use might be a problem.

- ✓ Ask yourself if you continue behaviors or using substances despite negative consequences.

- ✓ Recognize the biological signs and symptoms of addiction.

- ✓ Recognize the psychological signs and symptoms of addiction.

- ✓ Recognize the social signs and symptoms of addiction.

- ✓ Recognize the spiritual signs and symptoms of addiction.

Chapter 2

TALK ABOUT AN "A-HA" MOMENT!

Discovering Our Brain-Centered Approach to Recovery
How do you know unless you look?

Talk about an "a-ha!" moment—the day I was introduced to brain SPECT imaging changed my life forever, and it could change yours too. It was the Spring of 1991 and I was the medical director of a dual diagnosis (mixed substance abuse and psychiatric disorder) inpatient treatment unit at a psychiatric hospital in Fairfield, CA. I walked into our weekly grand rounds, a meeting in which doctors get together to listen to one of their colleagues present some new or relevant education.

In this particular meeting, Jack Paldi, MD, a nuclear medicine doctor and the chief of medicine at a nearby hospital, was discussing brain SPECT (single photon emission computed tomography) imaging. Brain SPECT imaging, as Dr. Paldi explained, offered a functional view of the brain. He said it basically gave us three pieces of information. It showed areas of the brain that worked well, areas that worked too hard, and areas that did not work hard enough. So, basically, it showed good activity in the brain, too little, or too much.

During the discussion, Dr. Paldi showed the doctors brain scans of people suffering from depression, schizophrenia, brain injuries, and dementia. The images of the interior workings of the brains of these people fascinated me. Even more intriguing to me were the before-and-after treatment scans, which clearly showed that with the proper treatment, the brain could heal and patients could have better lives. The light bulb went on in my brain—if you change your brain, you can change your life. I spent the entire hour mesmerized by the images. By contrast, most of my colleagues just didn't get it. Why was I the only one who saw the value in those compelling images?

Perhaps it was because I was already looking at the electrical activity of the brain using a technique called qEEG or quantitative electro-encephalogram. When I finished my psychiatric specialty training in child and adolescent psychiatry in 1987, I was then stationed at Fort Irwin in the Mojave Desert, where the Army tank divisions were taught to fight the Russians in the desert. The day I moved into my office, in an old World War II Quonset hut, it was 115 degrees outside. Our clinic was cooled by a noisy swamp cooler that caked dust around the whole office space.

One day, shortly after I arrived, while rooting around the cabinets in my new clinic, I found an old Autogen biofeedback temperature trainer. Biofeedback is a treatment technique that uses instruments to measure a person's individual physiology and through feedback teaches them to control it. The temperature trainer was very easy to use. It involved attaching a small thermister (thermometer) to a person's baby finger to measure hand temperature, and with some simple mental techniques I found that I could teach people to warm their hands and relax their whole bodies.

I was so impressed with the biofeedback results for decreasing our soldiers' stress levels that I applied for a $30,000 grant to bring state-of-the-art biofeedback equipment to Fort Irwin. The request was initially denied, but at the end of the fiscal year, the Army had money left over and decided to fund my project so they would not lose the funds in the budget for the following year. The training I took not only taught me about body biofeedback, but also about a new field called neurofeedback, which trains the brain to function more efficiently. By 1991 when I walked into Dr. Paldi's SPECT grand rounds lecture, I had already been looking at and changing people's brains. I had just never seen such stunningly beautiful and instructive brain images before.

32

I immediately thought about how the brain scans could help my patients in the dual diagnosis unit. I began scanning my patients and quickly discovered that substance abuse is terrible for the brain. It was one thing to see the troubled lives that result from drug abuse, it was quite another to see the toxic and damaged brains. I saw that marijuana, cocaine, methamphetamines, Vicodin, heroin, and alcohol all seriously impaired brain function. The worst brains of all? Those belonging to people who use inhalants.

The images showed very damaged brains, which correlated directly to the damaged lives, relationships, and physical health of my patients. The scans were so powerful that I started bringing them home to show them to my children and effectively induced anxiety disorders related to substance abuse in all of them. I am happy that none of them have had a problem with drugs or alcohol, despite having a significant family history of alcoholism on their mother's side.

The power of the images led me to develop and be part of a series of posters and videos on substance abuse. *The Truth About Drinking*, hosted by Leeza Gibbons, won an Emmy for best educational television in 1999. I also was part of HBO's special *Small Town Ecstasy* and wrote and produced a DVD called *Which Brain Do You Want?* that focuses on young adults and teens with substance abuse. The Amen Clinics poster, Which Brain Do You Want?, now hangs in over 75,000 schools, prisons, and drug treatment centers worldwide.

I was hooked on brain imaging within weeks of attending Dr. Paldi's lecture because I felt that it made me a better doctor. It gave me more information so that I could make better treatment decisions. Plus, many patients were shocked into stopping drug abuse by looking at their damaged brains. But my passion was met with skepticism in the psychiatric field. Many mental health professionals derided the use of brain scans as a tool in helping to diagnose or treat patients. It was a very frustrating first decade. I was called everything from a quack to a snake oil salesman to a charlatan. FOR WANTING TO ACTUALLY LOOK AT THE BRAIN!

I often wondered what we should call the people who were treating psychiatric illnesses without looking. Given that I am not shy, I was challenging my colleagues by asking questions such as, "Why does psychiatry remain the only medical specialty that never looks at the organ it treats? Can you imagine an emergency room physician diagnosing a broken arm without taking an X-ray? Or a cardiologist recommending bypass surgery without looking at your arteries?" As you can imagine I was not winning any popularity contests among my colleagues.

In both the mental health and addiction treatment fields, however, things are changing. My co-author David, for example, was one of the first addiction professionals to embrace the power of brain imaging and it has been a critical part of his approach to treatment for more than a decade. He has seen first-hand how this brain-centered approach to treatment helps people break free from their addictions. He knows that many of the traditional methods of dealing with addiction problems—"just say no," "drugs are evil," and "the war on drugs"—aren't working. That is because they don't get to the root of the problem, which lies in the brain.

Treatment centers are now beginning to take notice too. We work closely with scores of drug treatment centers, evaluating, scanning, and treating many of their patients. In 2009, Sierra Tucson, one of the world's most respected treatment centers for addictions and behavioral disorders, put a brain SPECT imaging camera in their facility. It now sends its patients' brain scans to us at the Amen Clinics for interpretation. The scans of substance abusers coming out of Sierra Tucson are some of the worst I have ever seen and serve as a reminder of the very first scans I did twenty years earlier on my patients in the dual diagnosis unit. In the nearly two decades since then, I have seen brain scans of severely depressed people, schizophrenics, and even serial killers, but it is the brains of substance abusers, football players, and boxers that show the most damage.

The good news is that the brains of substance abusers have the potential for some of the greatest improvement. The before-and-after scans often reveal a stunning level of recovery. No matter what you are addicted to—drugs, alcohol, smoking, or overeating—your brain can recover too.

Let me help you understand the many SPECT scans you will see in this book. Again, SPECT is a study that looks at blood flow and activity in the brain. The scans below are called our surface view. They show us areas of the brain that are healthy versus those that are low in activity. In this view we are looking at the top 45 percent of brain activity. Anything below this threshold looks like a hole or a dent. The holes do not represent actual physical holes in

Healthy Scan

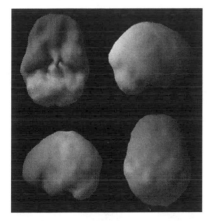

Alcohol Damaged Scan

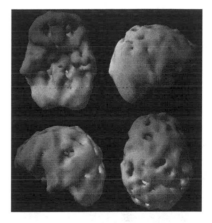

Cocaine Damaged Scan

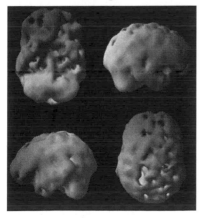

Inhalant Damaged Scan

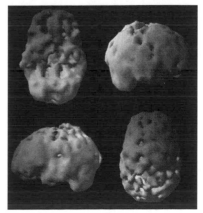

Meth Damaged Scan

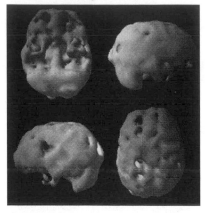

OxyContin Damaged Scan

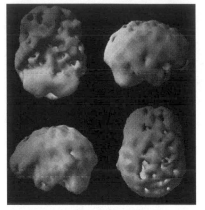

Xanax Damaged Scan

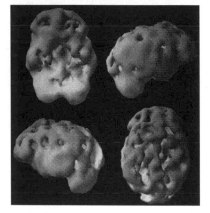

Vicodin Damaged Brain

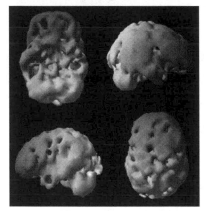

the brain, they represent areas that are low in activity. The healthy scan shows full, even, symmetrical activity. The drug- and alcohol-affected scans show generalized decreases in activity.

UNCHAIN YOUR BRAIN CHECKLIST

✓ SPECT brain imaging shows areas of the brain that work well, areas that work too hard, and areas that do not work hard enough.

✓ Biofeedback and neurofeedback train the body and brain to

work more efficiently.

✓ Marijuana, cocaine, methamphetamines, Vicodin, heroin, and alcohol seriously impair brain function.

✓ Of all drugs, inhalants do the most damage to brain function.

✓ Think about which brain you want—a healthy brain or a dysfunctional brain.

✓ Brain imaging can be beneficial in addiction treatment and has been adopted by Sierra Tucson.

✓ The brains of substance abusers have the potential for great improvement.

Chapter 3

HOW DO YOU KNOW
UNLESS YOU LOOK?

How Brain Imaging Takes Us Out of the 17th Century of Blame to Help Us Understand and Treat Addictions

Addiction is a brain disease. It doesn't mean you are a bad person.

A few years ago, I received a call from an attorney named John asking me if our brain imaging work could be of any help to one of his clients. He explained that his client, Joshua, had already been arrested ten times for violence, but he added that Joshua only got violent when he was drunk. John then told me about Joshua's latest run-in with the law. Joshua had been sober for six months when his girlfriend broke up with him. He couldn't handle the emotional stress of the breakup and went out and got drunk on a fifth of Peach Schnapps and a forty-ounce of St. Ides Malt Liquor.

Joshua then got into a car, drag raced his friend down the street, got into an accident, and left the scene of the accident. He flagged down a cab and drove around San Francisco for about half an hour. He thought, "I'm really in trouble now, so what the heck" and pulled a gun on the cabbie and stole $25 from him. The next morning, Joshua turned himself in.

His attorney told me that the prosecutor wanted to put Joshua away for eleven years. John asked if I would help him. I told him that I would do it, but only on two conditions:

1. Let me scan Joshua's brain.
2. Let me do a second brain scan while Joshua was drunk.

John laughed and said, "They don't let inmates get drunk!" I told him if he really wanted my help, he would have to find a way to work it out. A couple days later, John called and told me he couldn't believe it, but the judge had said, "Okay."

So we scanned Joshua while he was sober, and his brain scan showed a pattern we call the Ring of Fire, in which there is overall increased activity in the brain. Joshua came back a second time wearing his orange jumpsuit with shackles and leg irons, and I proceeded to get him drunk. I had gone to the liquor store earlier and had bought the exact same brands of alcohol he had been drinking that fateful night. So he started drinking the fifth of Peach Schnapps and the forty-ounce St. Ides Malt Liquor. About halfway through, he looked at me and with slurred speech, said, "This is the weirdest experience of my whole life. My doctor is getting me drunk while these two goons (the two police officers who had accompanied him) are watching."

Joshua's drunk scan showed a dramatic decrease in activity compared to his sober scan. There was low activity in his left temporal lobe, which is associated with violence. There was also low activity in his prefrontal cortex, which is the area associated with impulse control and planning, so he basically had no judgment.

The attorney, judge, and prosecutor came to my office to review the scans and reached a plea agreement. Joshua would have to serve three years in jail and then see an outpatient counselor every month for the next eight years. If he missed a single month, he would have to serve the whole eleven years in jail. The agreement addressed his responsibility for his actions but also took into account his illness. If we had never looked at his brain, we never would have known how much alcohol affected his behavior.

If you struggle with an addiction of any sort, you probably think it is because you are a bad, weak, or flawed person. After all, that is very likely the message you have been getting from the people around you.

"Why are you such a screw-up?"

"Why are you always letting me down?"

"Why can't you be more reliable?"

"Why can't you just stop?"

By the time you decide you need help and perhaps enter a treatment center or program, you likely feel like your addiction is all your fault or perhaps even that you deserve to be so miserable.

Brain imaging helps change these false and damaging notions. In working with thousands of substance abusers, David and I have found that brain imaging helps people realize that addiction is clearly a brain disease, not the result of a character flaw or personal weakness that can never be treated. David often tells people to think of addiction in the same way you would think of any other disease.

Take diabetes, for example, which is a disease of the pancreas that leads to problems with insulin and blood sugar regulation. Diabetes can lead to medical and behavioral consequences. With the proper treatment it can often be controlled so that diabetics can live a satisfying life. Similarly, addiction is a disease that can lead to health and behavior problems. With a brain-centered approach to treatment, addiction can often be controlled so you can lead a more productive and enjoyable life.

Realizing that addiction is a brain disease can be very powerful because it alleviates some of the stigma attached to substance abuse and bad behaviors. No longer do you have to feel like you are a bad person for having addictions or that the questionable behaviors you engage in while high or drunk define who you are.

That's the message David imparted to seventeen-year-old Nadine. When this teenager entered one of David's drug programs, she admitted that she felt like a loser because she would get drunk and then have sex with anyone. She was quick to label herself by saying, "I'm a slut." But when David asked her if she was also promiscuous when she was sober, she said no, she had never had sex with anyone when she was sober. After looking at the images of healthy brains and damaged brains, Nadine began to understand that her problems were not due to a character flaw, but to a brain problem. This helped her stop thinking of herself in such a negative and damaging way and gave her hope that she could change.

Realizing that addiction and substance abuse are brain diseases can also help parents understand that it isn't your fault if your child has an addiction. David routinely includes the entire family in his treatment plans and has found that parents of substance abusers often mercilessly beat themselves up over their child's problems.

"If only I had taken him to that Giants baseball game when he was seven instead of working, this wouldn't have happened. It's all my fault."

"If I had paid more attention to who she was hanging around with, I could have prevented this."

"I should have made him transfer to another school."

Parents often play the blame game with each other too.

"If you would have been home more often, you would have seen what was happening."

"You were always too lenient with her, letting her do whatever she wanted."

"You were so strict, you alienated him."

These thinking patterns are so detrimental to treatment and recovery. By contrast, focusing on addiction as a brain disease helps the entire family look at the brain as the organ that needs to be treated in order for the person with the addiction to get better.

41

Note that the concept of addiction as a brain disease does not relieve you of taking responsibility for your actions and behaviors. It gives you a better understanding of how your brain plays the central role in your addiction and how taking care of your brain is the key to breaking free from those addictions and behaviors that steal your life. In Chapter 4, we will go into much more detail about how addictions get stuck in your brain and how your behaviors can lead to addictions.

Brain Imaging Helps Identify Toxic Exposure

Arnie, fifty-six, came to the Amen Clinics with his wife who was seeking an evaluation for anxiety. She was very nervous about having a brain scan, so Arnie decided to get one too just as a way to calm her fears. When I saw Arnie's scan, it looked like his fifty-six-year-old brain was eighty-five years old. When I asked Arnie what he was doing to hurt his brain, Arnie thought for a moment and said, "Nothing."

After a few more minutes of asking about Arnie's daily habits to find out what could possibly make his brain look so bad, the subject of drinking came up. It turned out Arnie was having three or four drinks every day. He explained that as a business consultant, he spent a lot of time entertaining clients, taking them to dinner or out for drinks, so it was beneficial for his business. He never felt drunk or out of control so he didn't think it was a problem. That's when he had to be told that consuming that much alcohol on a daily basis was a BIG problem for his brain. Alcohol lowers overall brain function and decreases judgment, impulse control, memory, and motivation.

Healthy Scan   **Arnie's Alcohol Damaged Scan**

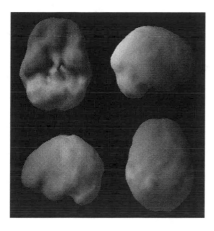 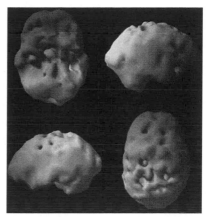

Arnie had no idea his daily drinking was harming his brain until he saw his scans. On a brain healthy plan that included abstinence from alcohol, regular exercise, mental exercise, vitamins, supplements, and fish oil, his brain improved greatly. A few months later, he wrote me saying he felt as mentally sharp as a twenty-year-old. His energy and memory had gotten a much-needed boost, and he felt smarter and more articulate. The changes had translated into increased revenues for his business and a host of lucrative new projects. He hadn't realized it, but his drinking had been holding him back.

Brain scans don't lie. Toxic exposure from alcohol—as in Arnie's case—drugs, nicotine, or excess caffeine can often clearly be seen on SPECT scans. These toxins can affect several important brain systems that play a major role in your ability to have the best life possible. Before we reveal how various substances affect your brain, it is important to gain some understanding about the brain systems that influence your behavior. Here is a quick crash course in the brain systems that run your life.

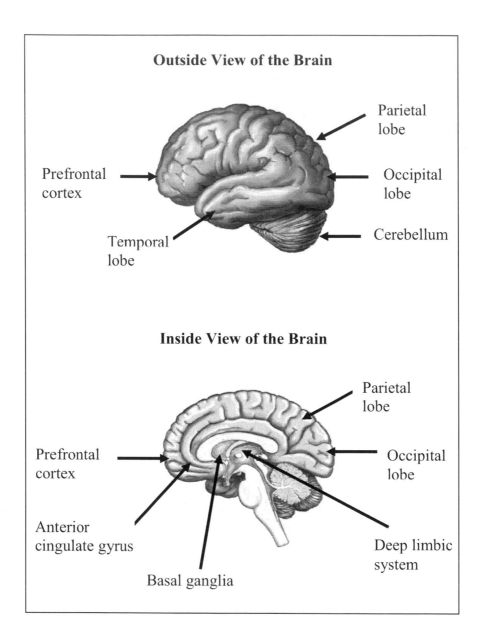

Outside View of the Brain

Parietal lobe

Prefrontal cortex

Occipital lobe

Temporal lobe

Cerebellum

Inside View of the Brain

Parietal lobe

Prefrontal cortex

Occipital lobe

Anterior cingulate gyrus

Deep limbic system

Basal ganglia

Prefrontal cortex (PFC): Think of the PFC as the CEO of your brain. Situated at the front third of your brain, it acts like a supervisor for the rest of your brain and body. It is involved with forethought, judgment, impulse control, planning, attention, follow through, empathy, and learning from the mistakes you make. When the PFC works well, it helps you say "no" to cocaine, marijuana, or chocolate pie. Low activity in the PFC is linked to a lack of clear goals, procrastination, a short attention span, bad judgment, impulsivity, and not learning from the mistakes you make, which makes you more likely to drink, smoke, or overeat. Alcohol lowers activity in the PFC, which is why people do such stupid things when they get drunk.

Anterior cingulate gyrus (ACG): I call the ACG the brain's gear shifter. It runs lengthwise through the deep parts of the frontal lobes and allows us to shift attention and be flexible and adaptable to change when needed. When there is too much activity in this area, you tend to become stuck on negative thoughts or actions, tend to worry, hold grudges, and be oppositional or argumentative. An overactive ACG may make you more vulnerable to being obsessive or to struggling with compulsive behaviors, such as gambling, eating disorders, or even working excessively.

Deep limbic system: Located near the center of the brain, the deep limbic system is involved in setting a person's emotional tone. When this area is less active, people tend to be more positive and hopeful. When it is overactive, negativity can take over and lower motivation and drive, decrease self-esteem, and increase feelings of guilt and helplessness. Abnormalities in the limbic brain have been associated with mood disorders, which set people up for addictions.

Basal ganglia: Surrounding the deep limbic system, the basal ganglia are involved with integrating thoughts, feelings, and movements. This part of the brain is also involved in setting a person's anxiety level. When there is too much activity in the basal ganglia, people tend to struggle with anxiety and physical stress symptoms, such as headaches, stomachaches, and muscle tension. High anxiety often sets up addictions. People drink to calm social anxiety, as described in David's case in the Introduction. They may overeat to settle their fears, or masturbate to relieve tension. With low activity in the basal ganglia, people tend to lack motivation. This area is also involved with feelings of pleasure and ecstasy.

45

Cocaine works in this part of the brain to release the pleasure chemical dopamine. Cookies, cakes, and other sugar-laden, fat-filled treats also activate this area, according to a fascinating book called *The End of Overeating* by Dr. David Kessler, the former commissioner of the U.S. Food and Drug Administration. Some trials suggest that sugar is actually MORE addictive than cocaine. For example, a 2007 study conducted by a team of French researchers found that when rats were allowed to choose between cocaine and water sweetened with either saccharin or sucrose, the vast majority of them (94 percent) chose the sweetened beverages over the cocaine. Not even increases in the doses of cocaine could lure the rats away from the sweet stuff.

Temporal lobes: The temporal lobes, located underneath your temples and behind your eyes, are involved with language, short-term memory, mood stability, and temper issues. They are part of the brain's "What Pathway," because they help you recognize and name "what" things are. Normal activity in this area generally results in stable moods and an even keel. Trouble in the temporal lobes often leads to memory problems, mood instability, and temper problems.

Parietal lobes: The parietal lobes toward the top back part of the brain are involved with sensory processing and direction sense. They are called the "Where Pathway" in the brain, because they help you know where things are in space, such as navigating your way to the kitchen at night in the dark. The parietal lobes have been implicated in eating disorders and self-body distortion syndromes, such as with anorexics who think they are fat. This is one of the first areas damaged by Alzheimer's disease, which is why people with this condition tend to get lost.

Occipital lobes: Located at the back of the brain, the occipital lobes are involved with vision and visual processing.

Cerebellum: Located at the back bottom part of the brain, the cerebellum is involved with physical coordination, thought coordination, and processing speed. There are large connections between the PFC and cerebellum, which is why many scientists think that the cerebellum is also associated with judgment and impulse control. When there are problems in the cerebellum, people tend to struggle with physical coordination, slow processing, and trouble learning. Alcohol is directly toxic to this part of the brain, which is why drunk people usually fail sobriety tests that involve balance and coordination moves like balancing on one leg or touching your fingertip to your nose. Improving the cerebellum through coordination exercises can improve your prefrontal cortex and also help your judgment.

Brief Brain System Summary

Prefrontal cortex—judgment, forethought, planning, and impulse control

Anterior cingulate gyrus—shifting attention

Deep limbic system—sets emotional tone, involved with mood and bonding

Basal ganglia—integrates thoughts, feelings, and movements, involved with pleasure

Temporal lobes—memory, mood stability, and temper issues, "what pathway"

Parietal lobes—sensory processing and direction sense, "where pathway"

Occipital lobes—vision and visual processing

Cerebellum—motor coordination, thought coordination, processing speed, and judgment

As seen on brain imaging scans, here are some of the ways addictive substances can harm your brain.

Drugs

All drugs of abuse appear to impair brain function. From my perspective, inhalants, opiates, and methamphetamine seem to be the worst drugs for your brain. Brains on these drugs look like Swiss cheese, with holes throughout indicating low brain activity. Opiates like heroin can cause temporary or permanent changes in the brain and alter brain chemistry, which may lead to mood swings, severe depression, anxiety, irritability, aggressiveness, sleep disturbances, and confusion, among other problems.

Methamphetamines decrease brain function and causes an array of problems, including memory loss, mood changes, depression, anxiety, paranoia, delusional thinking, and permanent psychological damage. In the group of eighty murderers we have scanned, half of them committed their crimes on methamphetamines. It is a very dangerous drug.

Cocaine use results in an array of cognitive problems according to a multi-year longitudinal study on rhesus monkeys exposed to the drug. The brain structure and function of rhesus monkeys is similar to that of humans, which makes them ideal test subjects for brain studies. The findings, presented at Neuroscience 2009, showed that the monkeys that used cocaine exhibited problems with memory, learning, planning, cognitive flexibility, and decision-making. Researchers noted that the errors the monkeys made during a series of cognitive tasks were similar to those made by people with attention deficit disorder (ADD), which may indicate that a shortened attention span and distractibility played a role.

Alcohol

Alcohol negatively affects the brain in a number of ways. It lowers overall blood flow and activity in the brain, which over time diminishes memory and judgment. A different study involving rhesus monkeys also presented at Neuroscience 2009 revealed that excessive alcohol consumption lowers the number of new brain cells that are formed in the hippocampus, one of the brain's main memory centers. In the study, monkeys that consumed alcohol experienced a 58 percent decline in the number of new brain cells formed and a 63 percent reduction in the survival rate of new brain cells.

Drinking large amounts of alcohol—four or more glasses of wine or the equivalent in hard liquor on a daily basis—raises the risk of dementia. New research shows that even moderate amounts of alcohol can have negative effects on the brain. A 2008 study appearing in the *Archives of Neurology* found that people who drink just one to seven drinks per week have smaller brains than nondrinkers, and those who have two or more drinks a day have even more brain shrinkage. When it comes to the brain, size matters!

Illegal drugs and alcohol aren't the only culprits. Everyday drugs like caffeine, nicotine, and excess sugar also compromise brain function.

Caffeine

Whether you get your caffeine from coffee, tea, energy drinks, or diet pills, it restricts blood flow to the brain, which lowers activity in the brain. It also dehydrates the brain, which makes it harder to think quickly and clearly. Caffeine also interferes with the sleep chemicals in the brain, which disrupts sleep patterns, leaving you feeling sluggish during the day. In addition, caffeine increases stress chemicals that stress your body and mind.

Nicotine

Found in cigarettes, cigars, chewing tobacco, nicotine patches, gums, and tablets, nicotine causes blood vessels to constrict, lowering blood flow to the brain. This deprives the brain of the nutrients it needs and eventually causes overall lowered activity. Smoking cigarettes is the number-one preventable cause of death claiming 500,000 lives a year.

Sugar

As I wrote in the Introduction, sugar is a drug that can be addicting. Consuming too much sugar causes your blood sugar to spike then plummet about thirty minutes later, leaving you feeling like you have brain fog. Low blood sugar levels are associated with lower overall blood flow to their brain. Sugar's toxic calories can also lead to obesity and excess inflammation, which increases the risk of developing type 2 diabetes, heart disease, and stroke—all of which are terrible for brain function. In some people, sugar can trigger seizure activity. A team of neurologists at Johns Hopkins University found that when children eliminated simple carbohydrates and refined sugar from their diet, it dramatically cut down on seizure activity, in some studies by more than half. Sugar can also promote mood disorders like depression and anxiety.

Jenny, twenty-six, had suffered from anxiety, depression, and fatigue for many years. She constantly craved sweets and would often experience headaches, mood swings, and dizziness throughout the day. When Jenny stopped eating treats made with refined sugar and gave up caffeine and alcohol, her symptoms disappeared.

Helping Break Denial

"Denial ain't just a river in Egypt" is a mantra often heard in 12-Step programs. That is because every person whose brain has been chained by addiction experiences denial. They are usually the last one to recognize that they have a problem. Most likely, you are no exception. You may be in denial yourself. You may have even told yourself one of the following statements in an attempt to convince yourself that you don't have a problem:

"I can quit smoking anytime I want. I just don't want to quit yet."

"I drink but I don't get drunk so it isn't a problem."

"I wouldn't drink so much if my wife wasn't so hard to live with."

"I'm passing most of my classes in school so my drug use can't be that bad."

"I only use drugs when I party, not every day."

"It isn't a big deal that I forgot to pick up my son because I was high. He found another ride home."

"I only binge eat when I get stressed out. Everybody does that."

After years of treating people with addictions, we have found that one of the best ways to break denial is to show someone an image of their brain. Chase, eighteen, is the son of a billionaire. He was drinking, smoking pot, taking OxyContin, and doing coke and meth, but was in complete denial about his addiction. His mother had tried to get Chase into treatment, but he resisted because he didn't think he had a problem. The mother saw my program on public television and asked if I would meet with her son. Brain scans were performed at the Amen Clinics and the images revealed that his brain was very toxic.

When Chase saw the images, he GOT IT immediately. Even though he felt like his drinking and drug use weren't a problem, the scan proved without a doubt that they were seriously harming his brain. Chase immediately cut out drinking and stopped doing drugs and has been clean and sober ever since. If he had never seen the pictures of his brain, he probably would still be in denial and continuing to abuse drugs and alcohol. It does not always happen so dramatically, but it does happen enough that I know the scans are often worthwhile.

Gilbert, a forty-six-year-old high-powered business executive, was using cocaine four to five times a week and drinking every day. He was very successful at work so he figured it wasn't bad for him. In fact, he thought it was *helping* him achieve his business goals by making him more sociable with clients and better able to put in long hours. When he looked at his brain, he exclaimed, "Oh my God! You have got to be kidding me. I have to change my life."

Motivating People to Follow a Treatment Plan

For many people, like Chase and Gilbert, seeing the images of their toxic brains is one of the greatest motivators for treatment. People are even more motivated to change their behaviors once they realize how important the brain is to their health, wealth, and happiness. Your brain is the organ of learning, loving, and living life to the fullest. Here are three of the basic principles about the brain that we both share with our patients to help motivate them to change.

Principle #1: Your brain is involved in everything you do.

Your brain controls how you think, feel, act, and interact. From the moment you wake up, it is your brain that plays the central role in your life. It is your brain that urges you to reach for that first morning cigarette or tells you to refrain from smoking. It is your brain that lets you stop drinking coffee after a single cup or pushes you to empty the whole pot. It is your brain that tells you to say, "no thank you" when your server asks you if you would like another glass of wine or allows you to order that second bottle of wine. It is your brain that pushes you away from the table or encourages you to reach for that third slice of chocolate cheesecake.

Your brain is involved in every decision you make. It also influences who you are and what you do: from social aptitude to athletic skills, parenting style to management approach at work, artistic talent to the type of music you like. Look at any aspect of behavior—from relationships, school, work, religion, and sports— and in the middle of all behavior is brain function. The impact of your brain affects your body too. Whether you live a long healthy life, suffer from a debilitating condition, or have your days cut short by a terrible disease, your brain is at the center of it all.

In fact, researchers from the University of Cambridge found that when people made bad decisions with their brains they took fourteen years off their lifespan. People who drank heavily, smoked, didn't exercise, and had poor diets at the age of sixty had the same risk of dying as someone with a healthy lifestyle who was seventy-four. The decisions your brain makes can steal or add many years to your life!

Principle #2: When your brain works right, you work right.

After looking at more than 57,000 brain scans, it has become clear to me that when your brain works right, you work right. A healthy brain makes it so much easier for you to be your best possible self, to be happier with your life, to be successful in your work, and to have loving relationships. When your brain is working at optimal levels, you are more likely to make good decisions, be reliable, and be an effective employee, friend, lover, parent, or child. Having a healthy brain also greatly increases your chances of sticking with a treatment program so you can overcome addiction.

Principle #3: When your brain is troubled, you have trouble in your life.

A troubled brain leads to trouble in your life. It is harder for you to be your best self or to achieve what you want out of life. Plus, you often act outside your own values, morals, and desires. Making poor choices and engaging in unhealthy behaviors are more common when your brain is not working at its best. With a troubled brain, it is much more challenging to follow a treatment plan, and even if you do manage to break free from your addictions, you are far more likely to relapse.

Years of analyzing brain images has led me to the concept that there is a difference between "will-driven behavior" and "brain-driven behavior." Will-driven behavior comes from a healthy brain. It allows you to exert conscious choice over a situation to work in your own best interest. Will-driven behavior is goal directed, productive, and helps you reach the goals you have set for your life. A damaged brain makes it much harder to control and direct behavior. It makes it more difficult to set goals and to plan and follow through on the actions necessary to achieve them.

An example of will-driven behavior is deciding to go to medical school, and then working diligently over time to make that happen, despite all of the various obstacles that get in your way. When your brain is not working right, you might dream of going to medical school, but you impulsively get high or drunk the night before your entrance exams. Then you don't perform well on the tests because you are hung over, and you do not get accepted to medical school.

When you understand these principles, you realize how critical it is to care for your brain so you can live the life you have always wanted. When people see images of the damage that drugs, alcohol, or other substances have done to their brain compared to scans of healthy brains, an exciting thing happens. They develop "brain envy." They want to have a better brain, and that motivates them to follow a treatment plan.

Helping to Identify Comorbid Conditions

We once treated a forty-two-year-old woman who had failed six alcohol treatment programs. She desperately wanted to stop drinking alcohol, but she couldn't follow through with any of the programs because she was so impulsive. She just couldn't say "no" whenever alcohol was around. Her brain scans showed severe damage to the PFC due to a head injury. It turned out that she had been kicked in the head by a horse when she was ten years old. She had no supervisor in her head. The PFC acts like the brain's brake, telling you to stop before engaging in detrimental behaviors. Without this internal supervisor, she constantly gave in to her cravings for alcohol. If we didn't address the damaged PFC, she would never be able to recover. Giving her a medication to enhance PFC function was very helpful to her and allowed her to follow through on an alcohol treatment program.

Brain Injury From Horse

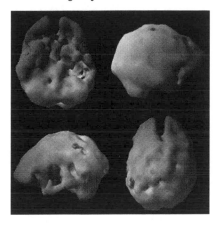

Randy, thirty-eight, was struggling with cocaine problems and had been arrested for domestic violence when he came to the Amen Clinics for help. He had already failed five other treatment programs and had convinced himself that he was just a terrible person and it was his own fault that he couldn't follow a program successfully. His brain scans told a different story. They showed very abnormal temporal lobe activity. Remember, the temporal lobes are involved in temper control. When Randy was placed on medication to improve temporal lobe function, he was finally able to stop using cocaine, he stopped being violent, and he became more reliable. Without treating the underlying brain dysfunction, Randy could have gone to one hundred treatment programs without success.

Many people with addictions are saddled with comorbid conditions—such as anxiety, depression, bipolar disorder, attention deficit disorder (ADD), or head injuries—all of which need to be treated in order to effectively help them be well. You can have the greatest treatment plan available or enter the most well-respected treatment center, but if you have underlying brain dysfunction, chances are you won't be able to follow through with the program. For lasting success, the brain problems must be treated in addition to the addiction. You will find out more about the link between mental health issues, brain injuries, and substance abuse in Chapter 5: The Four Pillars of Addiction and Healing.

Following Progress

There is no better way to find out if a treatment program is working than to see before-and-after images of the brain. Scans clearly show when a treatment plan is effectively healing the brain or when it needs to be adjusted. Thanks to imaging, we can make small changes to a person's program to promote even faster healing so it will be easier for you to break free from the addictions that steal your life. For patients, seeing the progress they have made can be a tremendous motivator to continue on the road to freedom from addiction. Even the slightest improvements in brain health can encourage you to stay on the right track.

Before Treatment Scan   **After Treatment Scan**

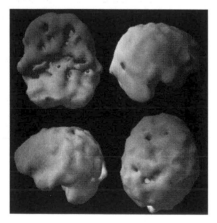
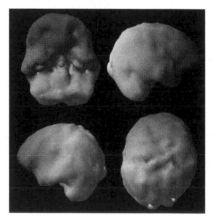

Prevention Education

Do you remember this old anti-drug commercial? It featured a man with a frying pan saying, "This is your brain," then cracking open an egg onto the hot skillet and saying, "This is your brain on drugs." This was a great attempt to show people how drugs affect your brain. With brain imaging, however, we can show what your brain really looks like on drugs, or alcohol, or nicotine, or caffeine. And it is not a pretty picture. These images can be extremely effective in making young people think twice before experimenting with damaging substances.

I have created a high school course called Making A Good Brain Great that is currently taught in more than three hundred schools in forty states and seven countries. The lesson plan includes showing students a number of scans of brains that have been damaged by drug or alcohol abuse. For many of the students, the images are so shocking that they choose to say "no" when someone offers them some pot, Vicodin, or alcohol. Independent research has shown the course increases pro-social attitudes in teenagers.

As part of a prevention education program, I created a DVD program called *Which Brain Do You Want?* It featured several teens with serious addictions talking about how they got addicted and how brain imaging helped them turn their lives around. One of the teens, Ian, revealed that he took a drag on his first cigarette when he was in the fifth grade. Within a few years, he was drinking alcohol, smoking pot, popping prescription pills like Valium, Xanax, Vicodin, and Percocet, taking mushrooms, dropping acid, and shooting heroin. Some of his friends used drugs when things got really tough at home or at school—if their parents were yelling at them a lot or if their girlfriend broke up with them. Ian didn't need a reason to use. It had become a habit for him, and he used all the time. He felt like the drugs were a way for him to escape. "Middle school is hard, high school is hard, growing up is hard," he said.

One night, he was so high that when he tried to take the two-and-a-half minute walk home from his friend's house, he ended up stumbling around with no sense of direction for about two hours. He couldn't find his house, and he couldn't figure out where he was. This was one of the events that made the teen start questioning his use of drugs and alcohol. Ian was slowly coming to the realization that escaping from your problems with drugs and alcohol doesn't mean you aren't creating new problems for yourself.

When Ian came to the Amen Clinics for a scan, he was very nervous to discover just how badly his drug and alcohol abuse had hurt his brain. As expected, his brain scan showed a lot of damage. "Is my brain stuck like that?" he asked. Fortunately, Ian learned that he could change his brain, and that if he stopped poisoning his brain with drugs and alcohol and adopted brain healthy habits, he could recover a lot of brain function. Since then, Ian has stopped abusing drugs and alcohol, and his brain and life are much better.

Also featured in the DVD, Carmelo was fourteen years old when he decided it would be cool to try taking drugs. He asked around at school and discovered that it was easy to find all kinds of drugs there—marijuana, Vicodin, Valium, cocaine, crystal methamphetamine, antidepressants, and Ecstasy, for example. He liked the way his first experience with drugs felt, and it made him want to do it again and do it more often. He started experimenting with all the different drugs he could find at school and started using more and more each day.

Drugs became the most important thing in Carmelo's life, and he found that he couldn't accomplish much of anything anymore. In fact, he didn't even finish high school. When Carmelo came to the Amen Clinics in his early twenties, he had started to think about what his life could have been like if he hadn't gotten hooked on drugs. If he had graduated high school and gone to college, he would be starting his career. Instead, he was stuck in a job that paid barely more than minimum wage. He was beginning to understand that all those school lectures he ignored about the dangers of doing drugs were true. And all the bad things they warned about in those lectures were now happening to him.

Carmelo's brain scan showed that his temporal lobes were inactive, which can contribute to moodiness, anger, difficulty reading, and poor social skills. After seeing his scan, Carmelo decided that he wanted a better brain and began changing his habits. Today, he's drug-free and doing great.

UNCHAIN YOUR BRAIN CHECKLIST

✓ Your brain is involved in everything you do.

✓ When your brain works right, you work right.

✓ When your brain has trouble, you have trouble in your life.

✓ The prefrontal cortex (PFC) is the CEO of your brain.

✓ The anterior cingulate gyrus (ACG) is the brain's gear shifter.

✓ The deep limbic system is involved in setting a person's emotional tone.

✓ The basal ganglia are involved in setting a person's anxiety level.

✓ The temporal lobes are involved with language, short-term memory, mood stability, and temper.

✓ The parietal lobes are involved with sensory processing and direction sense.

✓ The occipital lobes are involved with vision.

✓ The cerebellum is involved with physical coordination and thought processing.

✓ Brain imaging helps people realize that addiction is a brain disease, not a personal weakness.

✓ Brain imaging helps identify toxic exposure.

✓ Brain imaging helps break denial.

✓ Brain imaging helps motivate people to follow a treatment plan.

✓ Brain imaging helps identify comorbid conditions.

✓ Brain imaging helps follow progress.

✓ Brain imaging helps with prevention education.

Chapter 4

HOW ADDICTIONS GET STUCK IN YOUR BRAIN

And How to Get Them Unstuck

Lots of people will abuse substances and suffer adverse consequences and stop.

There is a subpopulation that will abuse substances, have adverse consequences, and then continue on in their patterned use of compulsions, loss of control, and continued use despite adverse consequences.

Jessica, twenty-three, had way too much to drink at her company holiday party and came on to the boss... in front of his wife! When she went back to work the next day, she got fired. Jessica felt humiliated and vowed never to get drunk again. And she didn't. She would still go out to bars with her friends, but she always stopped after a couple of drinks.

Robbie, twenty-five, went to his company's holiday party and got so trashed he went up to his supervisor and called her a bitch in front of the company CEO. Robbie got fired on the spot. The next night, he went out to a bar with a friend to "celebrate" the fact that he didn't have to work with that "bitch" anymore. He got drunk again and got a DUI when he drove home.

Derek, sixteen, was on the soccer team in high school. One day, he and his soccer teammates found a peephole to the girls' locker room where they saw the girls changing out of their clothes. A girl passing by outside noticed the group of guys, realized what they were doing, and turned them in to the school principal. Derek and his buddies got suspended for a week, and Derek never looked through the peephole again.

Brandon, forty-nine, was only fourteen years old when he peered threw an open window to sneak a peek at his sister coming out of the shower. He felt an incredible rush, but his sister caught him in the act, told their parents, and got Brandon into big trouble. The next day, though, all Brandon could think about was the strong arousal he felt from watching her, so later that day, he peered through his sister's bedroom window to watch her change clothes. He got caught again, and his parents grounded him for a month. Years later, Brandon placed a hidden camera in the bathroom of an apartment he was renting out so he could watch his female tenant in the shower. She found the camera and sued Brandon for $1 million, but even that didn't stop his voyeurism.

Tracy, forty-four, found out that her husband was having an affair and was so upset she decided to drown her sorrows in food. She went to the store and filled her cart with cupcakes, cheesecake, fudge brownies, and chocolate-covered pretzels. When she came home, she tore into the packages and stuffed them in her mouth. Within minutes of finishing her umpteen-thousand-calorie feast, she felt sick to her stomach. She spent most of the night throwing up, and the next day, she still felt queasy. She swore off bingeing and went back to her normal eating routine.

Stacey, thirty-six, started bingeing twenty years ago when she got cut from the high school drill team. She went home and ate everything she could find in the kitchen cupboards. The sickness that followed didn't deter her from doing it again when her boyfriend dumped her, when she didn't get into her first-choice college, or when she didn't land the job she wanted. Even the fact that she had gained thirty pounds and hated the way she looked couldn't keep her from bingeing whenever something bad or stressful happened in her life.

Why are some people who overdo it with alcohol, food, sex, or other things, able to remember the consequences of their actions, learn from their mistake, and avoid repeating the behavior? And why do others minimize the consequences, maximize the pleasure they got from the activity, and continue to engage in the same

destructive behavior? The answer lies in t̶
wired.

Why Am I A Slave to These Cravings? Unde
Brain's Reward System

Whether you experience consequences and quit   ...avior
or keep repeating it depends in large part on the biological makeup
of your brain and your brain's reward system. What is the brain's
reward system? It is an intricate network of brain systems and
neurotransmitters that are critical to human survival. It drives us to
seek out the things we need to stay alive and carry on the human
race.

For example, when we are hungry we are motivated to eat
because food tastes good, and it eliminates hunger and cravings.
Drinking water quenches our thirst and makes us feel cool and
refreshed. It is the same with sex. The physical pleasure we feel
from the sexual act drives us to repeat the behavior. The brain's
pleasure centers link to the emotional memory centers to create
powerful memories that drive us to repeat rewarding behaviors. If
we got no rewards from eating, drinking, or having sex, we
wouldn't be motivated to do them and we certainly wouldn't last
long on this planet.

Many other things that are not necessarily crucial to our
survival also activate the reward system, like listening to music,
taking a warm bath, or looking at a beautiful painting. Then there
are substances and behaviors that are actually detrimental to our
health and well-being that cause the reward system to kick into
high gear—cocaine, methamphetamines, heroin, alcohol, caramel
fudge brownies, playing video games, excessive texting, and
gambling, to name just a few.

Let's take a closer look at the neurotransmitters and brain
systems involved in the reward system so you can see how it works
and how it gets out of whack. First, let's examine the role played
by four neurotransmitters. Neurotransmitters act as the brain's

...rs, relaying information within the brain. The strength or ...ness of each of these neurotransmitters plays an important ...e in your ability to stop engaging in bad behaviors or in driving you to addiction.

Brain Chemicals Involved With Cravings And Self-Control

- Dopamine—motivation, saliency, drive, stimulant
- Serotonin—happy, anti-worry, calming
- GABA—inhibitory, calms, relaxes
- Endorphins—pleasure and pain-killing properties

Dopamine is a feel-good chemical. Whenever we do something enjoyable, it's like pressing a button in the brain to release a little bit of dopamine to make us feel pleasure. If we push these pleasure buttons too often or too strong, we reduce dopamine's effectiveness. Eventually, it takes more and more excitement and stimulation to feel anything at all. Cocaine, methamphetamines, alcohol, and nicotine all cause dopamine surges that make these substances highly desirable—sometimes even more desirable than the things we need to survive like food, water, and sex. The amount of dopamine released when drugs are taken can be two to ten times more than what your brain produces for natural rewards.

Drugs and alcohol aren't the only substances that can hijack your brain. Playing video games, gambling, and looking at Internet pornography can produce the same effect. So can certain foods. In *The End of Overeating*, Dr. David Kessler, a former FDA commissioner, writes that the high-fat, high-sugar combos found in many mouthwatering snacks light up the brain's dopamine pathway similar to the way drugs and alcohol do. He suggests that some people can actually get hooked on chocolate chip cookies the way other people get addicted to cocaine. Kessler and his team of researchers have seen this theory at work in animals, too. In one study, they found that rats will work increasingly hard for a high-fat, high-sugar milkshake, and that they will consume greater quantities of it if more sugar is added. The 2007 study I mentioned in Chapter 3 found that sugar is actually MORE addictive than cocaine.

The concept is simple. When we eat a bowl of fresh berries, our brains release small amounts of dopamine, which makes us feel good. When we eat things like caramel fudge brownies, our brains pump out lots of dopamine, which makes us feel *really* good. This increases the *saliency*, or the relative importance, of caramel fudge brownies in our minds. Soon we no longer get much pleasure from eating berries and begin craving caramel fudge brownies instead.

Exercise and green tea have been shown to be natural ways to increase dopamine in the brain.

Serotonin is thought of as the happy, anti-worry, flexibility chemical. Many of the current antidepressants work on this neurotransmitter. When serotonin levels are low, people tend to be worried, rigid, inflexible, oppositional and argumentative, and suffer with anxiety, depression, obsessive thinking, or compulsive behaviors. Serotonin is raised in the brain by its amino acid precursor, l-tryptophan. Amino acids are proteins. Unfortunately, l-tryptophan does not compete well against the other proteins to get into the brain. Exercise increases l-tryptophan in the brain because the other proteins go into the muscles thereby decreasing the competition for l-tryptophan to get into the brain. Simple carbohydrates increase l-tryptophan in the brain, which is why some people can get hooked on cookies, bread, potatoes, and sugar. We will talk a lot about the proper use of diet and exercise as a way to unchain your brain.

GABA, or gamma-aminobutyric acid, is an inhibitory neurotransmitter that calms or helps to relax the brain. If you have suffered an emotional trauma or you are under a lot of stress, GABA may be depleted and your emotional or limbic brain may become excessively active, making you feel anxious, uptight, or sad. This makes you eat or drink in an attempt to calm your limbic brain.

The amino acid supplement GABA can help, as can B6, magnesium, lemon balm, kava kava, and valerian.

Endorphins are the brain's own natural pleasure and pain-killing chemicals. They are the body's own natural morphine or heroin-like substances. These substances are heavily involved in addiction and the loss of control. Cocoa and dl-phenylalanine have been shown to increase endorphin production in the brain.

Now let's take a look at the brain systems that drive you to seek out rewarding behavior and that regulate your self-control.

Brain Systems Involved With Cravings And Self-Control

- Nucleus accumbens (basal ganglia)—pleasure and motivation center
- Deep limbic system—emotional memory centers, triggers of behavior
- Prefrontal cortex (PFC)—focus, judgment, and impulse control

Nucleus accumbens: Located deep within the brain in an area called the basal ganglia, the nucleus accumbens is the pleasure and motivation center of the brain. It is one of the primary drivers that trigger your behavior.

Deep limbic system: Lying deep inside your brain, the deep limbic system houses your brain's emotional memory centers and can drive you to action. According to my friend, addiction specialist Mark Laaser, PhD, the arousal template in the emotional memory centers of the brain underlies many behaviors that get out of control. It is important to understand where you were and how old you were when you experienced your first pleasurable or arousing experience. This intense emotionally pleasurable experience often lays the neural tracts for later addictions, even if the experience happened as early as age two or three. The first experience gets locked into the brain, and when you get older you seek to repeat the experience because it was the way you had the initial arousal or pleasurable experience, like the first time you tasted ice cream, fell in love, had sex, or used cocaine. Understanding the triggers for emotional eating, smoking, or drinking can be very helpful to breaking addictions.

Prefrontal cortex: The prefrontal cortex (PFC) is responsible for impulse control, judgment, focus, and follow through. It is the brain's brake, which reins in your actions and makes you stop and think before doing something you might regret. The PFC is larger in human beings than in any other animal. It is the part of the brain that makes you human. It represents 30 percent of the human brain. Compare that to 11 percent of a chimpanzee's brain, 7 percent of a dog's brain, and 3 percent of a cat's brain. Cats have little forethought and impulse control. The strength or weakness of this brain system determines in large part whether you can say "no" to temptations or give in to your cravings.

Why Can't I Just Say "No?" The Brain's Self-Control Circuit

The brain systems that drive you to seek out things that bring you pleasure and the PFC, which puts on the brakes when you are about to engage in risky behavior, work in concert to create your self-control circuit. In a healthy self-control circuit (see Figure 4.1), an effective PFC provides impulse control and good judgment while the deep limbic system offers an adequate dose of motivation so you can plan and follow through on your goals. Healthy dopamine levels drive you to pursue your passions and find your bliss in life while a healthy PFC acts as the reins or the brake so you do not get out of control. When these chemicals and brain areas are in balance, you can be focused, goal-oriented, and have control over your cravings. You can say "no" to alcohol, hot fudge sundaes, cigarettes, gambling, sex fetishes, and many other bad behaviors.

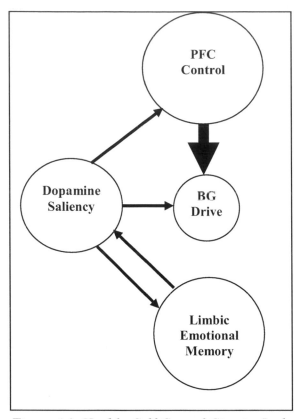

Figure 4.1: Healthy Self-Control Circuit. In the healthy self-control circuit, the prefrontal cortex (PFC) is strong and there is good balance between the chemical dopamine and the basal ganglia (BG), which houses the nucleus accumbens, and limbic or emotional circuits in the brain.

In the addicted brain, the PFC is diminished and the drive circuits take control. When the PFC is underactive (see Figure 4.2), it can create an imbalance with the reward system and cause you to lose control over your behavior. When this is the case you are more likely to fall victim to your cravings. Having low activity in the PFC often results in a tendency for impulse-control problems and poor internal supervision.

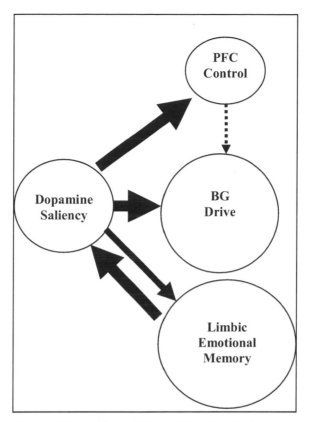

Figure 4.2: Addicted Drive Circuit. In the addicted circuit, the PFC is weak, so it has little control over unbridled passions that drive behaviors. Addiction actually changes the brain in a negative way making it harder to apply the brakes to harmful behaviors. In the non-addicted brain, the PFC is constantly assessing the value of incoming information and the appropriateness of the planned response, applying the brakes or inhibitory control as needed. In the addicted brain, this control circuit becomes impaired through drug abuse, ADD, sleep deprivation, or a brain injury, losing much of its inhibitory power over the circuits that drive response to stimuli deemed salient.

Researchers have been studying addicted drive circuits in the brains of substance abusers for many years. Thanks to brain imaging, they are now seeing similar brain patterns in people with other bad behaviors, including behavioral addictions, such as gambling, sex, and overeating. For example, researchers at Brookhaven National Laboratory have been using PET brain imaging to conduct a series of studies on the inner workings of the brain's self-control circuit in obese patients. The scans reveal the same patterns of brain dysfunction found in people addicted to cocaine or alcohol. Other PET studies from this same team show a correlation between a higher body mass index (BMI) and decreased activity in the PFC, which means overweight and obese people are likely to have less self-control.

Anything that decreases activity to the brain robs you of good judgment and makes you more likely to give in to your cravings. Pushing on your brain's pleasure buttons too hard or too often can cause the brain's brakes to fail by decreasing activity in the PFC. Poor sleep, attention deficit disorder (ADD), and head injuries are also associated with reduced PFC activity. Many people don't even realize they have had a head injury that has affected their self-control.

Jason, who had Tourette's Syndrome, came to the Amen Clinics for an evaluation for a substance abuse problem. He was in withdrawal and pretty irritable during our testing. The Tourette's caused him to have a head tic. In order to have a good quality scan, it is important to lie perfectly still in the SPECT camera for fifteen minutes. But his tic was definitely interfering with his ability to be still. In order to help him, I climbed on top of him and held his head still for the fifteen-minute test.

His SPECT scans revealed that he likely had a brain injury to his left frontal and temporal lobe. When I asked him if he had ever suffered a head injury, he said, "Fuck no!"

Sometimes people with Tourette's have what is called corprolalia, or involuntary swearing. Although I was not sure it was involuntary in Jason's case. Jason had been asked about brain injuries five times by our historian and was tired of saying "no." But, as we have seen, people often forget about important brain injuries and need to be asked many different times, especially if we see evidence on their scans. When he said no again, I asked if he was sure.

"Fuck no!" This time with more irritation and emphasis.

I persisted. "Did you fall out of a tree?"

"Fuck no!"

"A sports injury?"

"Fuck no!"

"A car accident?"

"Fuck no!"

Then Jason's face changed, which is a right-hemisphere phenomenon. The right side of the brain lights up when we have an "a-ha" moment. He looked at me and said, "Does a motorcycle accident count?"

I asked what happened and he went on to explain that he had been riding his motorcycle around a lake when a deer came out into the middle of the road. He didn't want to hit the deer so he spilled his bike onto his left side and broke his left jaw. He said, "Does that count?"

"Fuck yes," I replied. "Of course, that counts!"

Adolescents typically have less efficient activity in the PFC because this part of the brain isn't fully developed until about age twenty-five. Until that age the brain is undergoing a crucial development process called myelinization, in which a protective substance called myelin wraps around the brain's neurons. Myelinization helps the brain's nerve cells work up to ten to one hundred times more efficiently, and it starts at the back of the brain during infancy and works its way forward to the PFC during adolescence and young adulthood.

Until the process is complete, a young adult's brain isn't fully mature and it lacks some of the developmental wiring that carries the "stop" messages to the rest of the brain. Because of this adolescent brains may not be capable of fully comprehending the consequences of risky behavior. Just think back to your own youth. Were you as mature at age seventeen as you were at twenty-five? David and I both needed some time to develop maturity. Some days I know I am still working on it.

Because their brains' brakes are still developing, adolescents are particularly vulnerable to addiction. And those addictions may cause changes in the way the brain works and responds to rewards and consequences. This is why it is so important for young people to prevent addictions in the first place.

People at the other end of the age range are also at risk for decreased activity in the PFC. Coronary artery surgery and frontal lobe dementia, which affects seniors, can take the PFC offline, allowing the limbic brain to take over. Some medications can also damage your brain's self-control circuit and make you more likely to be impulsive or engage in compulsive behaviors.

That is exactly what Gary Charbonneau claims happened to him. According to newspaper reports, Charbonneau, who has Parkinson's disease, claims that when he started taking the drug Mirapex to control the tremors associated with the condition, he started gambling compulsively and lost $260,000. He sued the makers of the drug and was awarded more than $8 million in a settlement.

How could a Parkinson's drug turn someone into a compulsive gambler? Here's a look at the neuroscience behind Charbonneau's claims. Parkinson's occurs due to a lack of dopamine in areas of the brain involved with movement and coordination. Mirapex, like other drugs used to treat Parkinson's disease and restless leg syndrome, is a dopamine agonist, which means it activates dopamine. It effectively activates dopamine in the movement and coordination centers of the brain to provide relief from tremors, but it also increases the release of dopamine in the pleasure centers of the brain.

According to dozens of studies, this can lead to impulsive and compulsive behaviors, such as gambling, shopping, binge eating, and hypersexuality. A 2009 study appearing in *Mayo Clinic Proceedings* and involving 267 Parkinson's patients found that new-onset compulsive gambling or hypersexuality occurred in more than 18 percent of patients taking dopamine agonists.

Having low blood sugar levels also reduces PFC activity. In a 2007 article, Matthew Gailliot and Roy Baumeister outline the critical nature of blood sugar levels and self-control. They write that self-control failures are more likely to occur when blood sugar is low. Low blood sugar levels can make you feel hungry, irritable, or anxious—all of which make you more likely to make poor choices. Many everyday behaviors can cause dips in blood sugar levels, including drinking alcohol, skipping meals, and consuming sugary snacks or beverages, which causes an initial spike in blood sugar then a crash about thirty minutes later.

In some cases, the very behaviors you want to quit—such as drinking alcohol, taking drugs, or eating high-carbohydrate foods like white bread, pasta, or muffins—make it harder for you to stop because they decrease activity in the PFC. Even though the goal would be to stop drinking, hold the cigarettes, or maintain a healthy weight, you do not have the willpower (or the PFC power) to say "no" on a regular basis. For example, a 2009 study out of the University of Pittsburgh found that when you crave a cigarette, it decreases your brain's ability to stay focused, which lowers your ability to exercise self-control and increases your odds of reaching for that cigarette.

There is no doubt that when people get drunk, they tend to do stupid things. That is because alcohol reduces activity in the PFC, making you more impulsive. A team of addiction researchers has discovered that impaired judgment from drinking continues during the morning-after hangover period. Writing in a 2010 issue of the journal *Alcohol, Clinical and Experimental Research*, the team reported that people who drink to intoxication show a reduced ability to concentrate and make accurate decisions while hungover.

The Addict's Dilemma

1. Your prefrontal cortex tells you that you need to stop your behavior.

2. Your pleasure centers override those commands with uncontrollable cravings.

3. The things you crave decrease function in your PFC, robbing you of the willpower to follow through on your plans to quit.

Things That Lower PFC Activity And Make You More Vulnerable To Addictions

- Poor sleep
- Head injuries
- ADD
- Being under the age of twenty-five
- Coronary artery surgery
- Frontal lobe dementia
- Medications
- Smoking
- Caffeine
- Alcohol
- Drugs
- Sugar-filled treats
- High-carbohydrate foods
- Low blood sugar levels

*Addictions occur when the drive circuits hijack the
brain and take control.*

When the reward system takes over, signals from the reward system to the PFC are disrupted and you do stupid things. It is like you are living without any forethought—like a cat. Allan, the son of a friend of mine, lost his job due to alcohol. His wife was sick and tired of his drinking and gave him an ultimatum—either go to Alcoholics Anonymous (AA) or move out. Desperate to save his marriage, Allan promised to join an AA group. On his way to his first AA meeting, however, he passed by a bar and impulsively went inside and proceeded to get drunk. He came home at 2 a.m. and wasn't wearing any pants. As you can imagine, this didn't go over well with his wife, and his whole world crashed after that.

Your brain systems either help or hurt your self-control. Your PFC is involved in making the moment-by-moment decisions that determine your behavior. It also plays out the consequences of your potential decisions, and then decides whether or not to take action. For example, my co-author David went to a Bob Dylan concert and someone sitting next to him lit up a bong. The smell of pot wafting his way sparked cravings that David still struggles with to this day. David thought about how he would love to take a hit off that bong, but his PFC—strengthened by years of being drug-free—played out the consequences in his mind. "If I take a hit, it will lower my impulse control and make me want to do other drugs, too. Then I am likely to relapse, and it will be harder for me to quit." After going through the scenario, David simply got up and moved so he couldn't see or smell the bong. If he had been drunk, his PFC activity might have been reduced and he might not have been able to resist the lure of that bong.

*Once you cross the line to addiction, you can't go back to
controlled use.*

Abusing drugs, alcohol, food, or any other substance changes your brain's reward system. This is why people with addictions can't go to treatment centers, AA meetings, or weight-loss clinics to stabilize their life and then return home and use drugs casually, drink a glass of wine with dinner, or treat themselves to an occasional food binge.

Kasey, sixteen, went into treatment for heroin addiction. She stayed clean during the treatment process and by the time she went home, she felt like she was "cured." She was so certain that she had kicked her heroin habit that she thought it would be okay to take a few prescription pain pills to take the edge off when she got back home. Her brain instantly recognized the opiates in the painkillers and that brought back the intense cravings for heroin. Within a few weeks, Kasey's dad found black tar heroin in her purse and sent her back to a treatment facility.

Many people use drugs, alcohol, food, and other substances or behaviors as a way to self-medicate imbalanced brains.

Soon after starting our brain imaging work it was very clear that many people use drugs, alcohol, food, and other substances or behaviors as a way to self-medicate imbalanced brains. For example, when some areas of the brain are underactive, people may turn to stimulants—such as cocaine, methamphetamine, or caffeine—to stimulate the brain. People who have overactive brain systems may use downers—such as alcohol, marijuana, sedatives, painkillers, and high-carbohydrate snacks and sweets—to calm the brain.

MIT researchers demonstrated that simple carbohydrates, such as cookies or candy, boost serotonin levels, which explains why some people eat when they are worried or under a lot of stress. Although these substances may appear to achieve the desired effect on a short-term basis, they damage the brain's reward system and your ability to control your behavior.

When you stop the bad behaviors, your brain can create new pathways between the reward system and the PFC. This is not irreversible brain damage.

There is no question that addictions harm the brain, but the most important thing to understand is that your brain can heal. If you stop your bad habits, you can improve your brain function and increase your ability to maintain self-control so you can break free from your addictions. In Part Two, you will discover many simple strategies to strengthen your PFC to improve your self-control. In addition, you will find ways to balance the neurotransmitters and brain systems of the reward system so you can gain control over your behavior.

The Addiction Cycle and the Four C's

The descent into addiction follows a well-established pattern that is characterized by the four C's:

1. Craving
2. Compulsion
3. Loss of control
4. Continued use in spite of consequences

Each of these steps to addiction is associated with certain brain dysfunctions. Cravings are the result of high levels of dopamine or endorphins being released whenever you take the substance or engage in that particular behavior. Low serotonin levels make it hard for you to feel pleasure from anything else and you feel compelled to chase the feeling or the high. When you lose control over your behavior, it often involves an underactive PFC. Continuing to use in the face of consequences is often triggered by your brain's emotional memory centers.

Let's take a look at how these four steps played out for James, a pathological gambler.

Craving. James still remembers the first time he ever stepped foot in a casino. He was thirty-one and it was his friend's bachelor party. The guys had decided to get high on cocaine and then hit the blackjack tables. James was winning big that night and felt an incredible rush of excitement. After a couple of hours, the other guys left to go to a strip club, but James wanted to play another hand, then another, then another.

He stayed at that table all night. Every time he won a hand, his brain was releasing dopamine, which gave him an intense feeling of pleasure. The more he played, the more he wanted to play. When James returned home, he kept remembering how great he felt at the blackjack table, and he wanted that feeling again ... badly. He started going to the casino regularly, getting high on cocaine and gambling away his money.

Compulsion. The surges in dopamine while gambling effectively reduced his ability to feel pleasure from natural things. It lowered his serotonin levels, which made his life seem dull and boring anytime he wasn't gambling. His brain no longer felt right without the reward, and he felt compelled to gamble just to relieve the discomfort.

Loss of control. James was gambling so much that he was losing all his money. He blew through his savings and needed money for rent or he was going to get evicted. He impulsively wrote a bad check just so he could pay his bills, but instead of paying the bills he took that money and gambled it away. This lack of judgment and impulsiveness indicated that his brain's PFC likely had lowered activity and could no longer rein in his behavior.

Continued use in spite of consequences. Realizing he was in trouble, James tried to stop gambling. He could keep himself under control until he saw a TV ad for a local casino, saw a red carpet like the one at the casino, or saw his nephew playing a card game with a friend. His brain's emotional memory centers—the hippocampus, amygdala, and nucleus accumbens—turned on his cravings any time he saw anything that reminded him of gambling. His landlord eventually threw him out, and James had to sleep on the couch at a friend's apartment, but even though he lost his apartment he kept gambling.

No matter what you become a slave to—drugs, alcohol, chocolate, shopping, gambling, video games, caffeine—the brain follows the same cycle to addiction. Getting your brain unstuck will require you to take control back over your brain, by enhancing your prefrontal cortex and balancing the systems and neurotransmitters that run your life.

UNCHAIN YOUR BRAIN CHECKLIST

- ✓ Doing enjoyable things releases dopamine, a feel-good chemical, in the brain.

- ✓ Drugs and alcohol; high-fat, high-sugar, high-salt foods; and thrilling behaviors can release large amounts of dopamine.

- ✓ Neuronal pathways link the brain's pleasure centers to its emotional memory centers to create powerful memories and make rewarding behaviors more salient.

- ✓ In a healthy self-control circuit, the PFC is strong and there is good balance between the brain's pleasure centers and emotional centers.

- ✓ Addictions occur when the drive circuits hijack the brain and take control.

- ✓ Decreased activity in the PFC increases impulse control problems.

- ✓ The things you crave can lower activity in the PFC and reduce impulse control, keeping you chained to your addiction.

- ✓ You can rewire your brain to create a healthier self-control circuit.

- ✓ The addiction cycle is characterized by the four Cs: craving, compulsion, loss of control, and continued use in spite of consequences.

Chapter 5

HOW DID I GET
THIS WAY?

The Four Pillars of Addiction and Healing

Simple answers are not sufficient. It's never just one thing.

Maria, forty-seven, had always enjoyed a couple of glasses of wine with dinner. The mother of three felt it helped her relax after a busy day shuttling the kids to school, soccer practice, tutoring sessions, and piano lessons. When Maria turned forty-nine, her mother-in-law was diagnosed with Alzheimer's disease and moved in with the family. That's when Maria started having a glass of wine while she prepared the evening meal and then another couple glasses with her meal. Over time, she noticed that almost the entire bottle would be gone before she finished making dinner and then she would polish off another half bottle or more with dinner. She never felt drunk or out of control so she didn't see it as a problem. When her husband expressed concerned about her drinking, Maria admitted she was drinking more than she used to but blamed it on the added stress of having her mother-in-law in the house.

Rita, thirty-three, hated the way she looked. Since high school she had been a binge eater, and the late-night refrigerator raids had added about ten pounds a year to her five-foot-three-inch frame bringing her to her current weight of 270 pounds. But Rita didn't feel like there was anything she could do about her weight—after all, nearly all of her relatives were obese. "It's my genetics," Rita would tell herself. "I'm doomed to be fat forever."

R.J., twenty, wanted to get into the best law school, but his grades at college weren't quite good enough so he started taking his friend's ADD medication Adderall to help him focus and be more alert. It allowed him to stay up all night, and his grades improved. But the drug gave him the jitters and he eventually started taking prescription sleeping medication or drinking excessively when he wanted to calm down. Eventually he was hooked and blamed law school requirements for his addiction.

Jake, thirty-seven, owned a large Internet company when he came to the Amen Clinics for addiction to alcohol and cocaine. Jake had always been focused on making money... and lots of it. It was the only thing he lived for. When his company took a downturn when the economy slumped, he felt like a failure and turned to cocaine and alcohol. The hard-charging entrepreneur was certain that his financial problems were the cause of his addiction.

Maria, Rita, R.J., and Jake all have something in common besides having addictions. They were all searching for simple answers to explain why they had become enslaved to their behavior. But when it comes to addiction, there usually are not simple answers. Rarely can we blame addiction on one thing. There are usually a number of factors involved.

For Maria, the problem wasn't just her mother-in-law. Her husband had just been diagnosed with a recurrence of cancer, her mother was getting a divorce, and her best friend had a brain tumor. Plus, she had started experiencing the effects of perimenopause—hot flashes, night sweats, and fluctuating hormones that increased her feelings of anxiety and irritability.

In Rita's case, genetics weren't the sole reason for her weight issues. Lying to herself about why she had been binge-eating for fifteen years was a big part of the problem. Low self-esteem, low thyroid levels, and sexual abuse when she was a teenager also contributed to the problem.

R.J. blamed his addiction on the fact that he needed to get better grades to get into the law school he wanted to attend. But the fact was that many other social and work obligations were taking too much time away from his schoolwork. He spent about thirty hours a week working as the editor of his college newspaper, devoted at least fifteen hours a week to a student political organization, was taking a double class load in an effort to graduate in three years instead of four, was dating three different girls, and liked going partying all night with his fraternity brothers. In addition, he was trying to live up to his parents' expectations and follow in the footsteps of his older brother who had gotten accepted to the top law school. All of these things played a part in his addiction.

Being financially strained wasn't the only reason Jake had turned to drugs and alcohol. He had a family history of alcoholism, slept only a few hours a night, drank diet sodas all day, grew up in a family with a lot of emotional distance, and had no sense of meaning or purpose beyond making money. His addiction resulted from the combination of all these contributing factors.

After working with thousands of patients, we have discovered that there are usually many combined biological, psychological, social, and spiritual factors that lead to addiction. For example, you may have heightened vulnerability due to a family history of addiction, then you fall off your bike as a child and suffer a head injury, and grow up with some sexual abuse as a teenager. Then as an adult, when your boss starts dumping extra projects on your desk, your child starts having trouble in school, and your savings are wiped out in the bad economy, it finally pushes you over the edge into addiction.

In order to understand and successfully treat addiction, it is best to take a bio-psycho-social-spiritual approach. This all-encompassing approach addresses all of the biological conditions, psychological issues, social influences, and spiritual factors that may be contributing to addiction. This approach is the most comprehensive, yet easiest, way to think about understanding and treating any addiction problem, any other mental health issue, or any medical condition for that matter.

Just think about diabetes. It involves biological conditions, such as a family history for the disease that makes you more vulnerable to it. There are psychological issues at play, including lying to yourself about your risk: "I'm only twenty-five. I'm too young to get diabetes." Social influences can drive you to engage in behaviors that increase your odds of getting the disease or preventing you from keeping it under control. For example, if your mom gets insulted if you say "no" to second and third helpings of her famous beef lasagna and chocolate mousse cheesecake, it makes you more likely to indulge in foods that are not diabetic-friendly. Lastly, spiritual factors—having a sense of meaning and purpose in your life—are more important than you might realize. If you don't feel like your life matters, then why take care of yourself to control your diabetes?

As with diabetes, all four of these areas come into play with addiction. In order to understand why you are addicted and to break free from your addictions, you must address all four pillars. You must look at the underlying *biology* of the problems, as well as your *psychology* or mind set, the *social* situation you find yourself in, and your *spiritual* beliefs. If you miss any of them, you will not be able to heal effectively. In this chapter, we will show you how each of these factors can contribute to the problem of addiction and how the path to healing lies within these four pillars.

The Amen Clinics 8 Circles Of Health And Healing

Understanding The Problem

BIOLOGY   PSYCHOLOGY

Brain function   How we talk to ourselves
   Blood flow (SPECT)   Self concept
   Electrical activity (qEEG)   Body image
Trauma/injuries   Upbringing
Allergies (food, mold, pet hair)   Developmental issues
Toxins (environment (mold), drugs,   Past emotional trauma
alcohol, excessive caffeine, smoking)   Past successes
Infections   Past failures
Genetics—family history   Grief
Physical illness—thyroid, fatty   Generational histories and
acid level, nutrient status   issues (immigrants, survivors
Hormones   of trauma, children/grand-
Nutrition   children of alcoholics)
Exercise   Hope
Sleep   Sense of worth
Medication   Sense of power or control
Dehydration

Quality of current environment   Sense of meaning & purpose
Connection to family, friends,   (Why does my life matter?)
community   Connection to higher power
Pets   (Who am I accountable to?
Stresses   What happens after I die?)
Relationships   Connection to past generations
Health   Connection to future generations
Finances   Connection to the planet
Work, school   Morality
Thrilling behavior   Values
Current successes or failures
Information

SOCIAL   SPIRITUAL

84

Healing Your Brain And Your Life

BIOLOGY

PSYCHOLOGY

Optimizing brain function
Protecting brain from trauma
Avoiding toxins (drugs, much
alcohol, nicotine, much caffeine,
food, or environmental allergens)
Healthy sleep
Treating any physical illness
Treating any psychiatric illnesses
Brain healthy diet
Exercise
Eliminate unnecessary meds
Neurofeedback, alpha stim
Supplements
Medications
Hyperbaric oxygen
Bright light therapy
Meditation/hypnosis

Understanding your
brain leads to forgiveness
ANT therapy (questioning
and correcting your thoughts)
History of your family
Life therapy—going through
each year of your life, working
through issues
Gratitude
Healing past emotional traumas
(EMDR)
Hypnosis/meditation
Offering hope
Clearly written goals to stay
on track

Optimizing the environment
Keeping you safe
Improving relationships and
community connections
Stress management techniques
Problem solving techniques
Work or school accommodations
Hope for the future
Opportunities
Information/education
Options

Discovering a sense of
meaning and purpose
(Why does my life matter?)
Evaluating your connection
to higher power (Who am
I accountable to? What
happens after I die?)
Explore connection to past
generations
Explore connection to future
generations and the planet
Define your morality
Clarify your values

SOCIAL

SPIRITUAL

Biological Factors That Make You More Vulnerable to Addiction

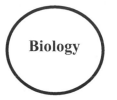

Your biological makeup and the health of your brain and body can either drive you to give in to your temptations or provide you with good judgment and stronger willpower. In regards to *biology*, we need to look at brain function, genetics, physical health, and the dietary issues underlying your addiction. Understanding what may be contributing to your problem is key to learning how to recover from your addictions.

Brain Function

The way your brain is wired and its overall health play a primary role in addiction. When your brain works right, you work right and are better able to resist temptations. When your brain is troubled, you are more likely to have trouble with addictions. There can be many reasons why your brain isn't functioning optimally, including head injuries, blood flow problems, allergies, and exposure to environmental toxins.

Genetics

Your family history matters. According to the National Institute on Drug Abuse, genetic factors account for 40 to 60 percent of a person's vulnerability to addiction. With early onset addiction prior to the age of fifteen, it is commonly 60 percent genetic, 40 percent environmental. When addictions set in later in life, genetic factors often play a smaller role. Remember that genetics is only part of the problem. Trying to blame your addiction solely on your genetic makeup will jeopardize your recovery.

Medical Conditions and Medications

When your body isn't healthy, it takes a toll on your brain, which can raise your risk for addiction. Conditions that cause chronic pain, such as fibromyalgia, cause changes in the brain and can lead to dependence on prescription painkillers as well as other unhealthy coping mechanisms. Having severe PMS, chronic fatigue syndrome, and many other conditions can also impact brain function and influence your habits. Low blood sugar is another problematic condition because it decreases brain activity and effectively lowers your ability to say "no" to unhealthy substances and behaviors. Hormonal imbalances can wreak havoc with brain function and leave you more vulnerable to addiction. You also need to be aware of the prescription medications you are taking. A number of medications can affect brain function in a negative way and increase your odds for addiction.

Poor Nutrition

You are what you eat… and drink! If you eat a junk-food diet, you will have a junk-food brain that increases your risk for addiction. You are also more likely to be overweight or obese. For some people, putting on too many pounds leads to taking diet pills or speed to suppress the appetite. Then they may feel the need to drink alcohol to calm the effects of the stimulants. It is a vicious cycle.

What your mother ate while she was pregnant with you matters, too. If your mom didn't consume adequate amounts of omega-3 fatty acids during pregnancy, then your brain suffers for it. Omega-3 fatty acids, found in foods like wild salmon, avocados, and walnuts, are rich in a type of fat called DHA. Why is that important for brain function? Did you know that 60 percent of the solid weight of your brain is fat, and a significant amount of the fat in your brain is DHA? Without enough of it, your brain can't develop or function normally.

Lack of Exercise

Lack of physical exercise negatively affects blood flow in the body, and subsequently to the brain. Low blood flow equals low activity, which equals lowered self-control. In a fascinating study that was published in a 2006 issue of *Pediatrics*, researchers found that teens who avoided exercise and instead spent a lot of time watching TV or playing video games tended to be at higher risk for risky behaviors like drinking, smoking, and doing drugs.

Lack of Sleep

Skimping on sleep is terrible for your brain function. Getting less than six hours of sleep a night has been associated with lower overall brain activity, which can affect your judgment, thinking, and self-control.

Psychological Factors That Make You More Vulnerable to Addiction

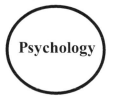

From a *psychological* standpoint it is important to look at how you are shaped by your thinking patterns and past experiences. Negative psychological factors may drive you to seek solace in unhealthy substances or behaviors. Some of the many psychological issues at play include how you talk to yourself, any past emotional trauma, past successes and failures, and your upbringing, self-image, and outlook on life.

How You Talk to Yourself

The way you talk to yourself can keep your brain chained or help you break free from addiction. Negative thinking cause negative brain changes that keep you trapped in your bad behaviors. Chapter 12: Kill the Addiction ANTs explores this notion in detail.

Past Emotional Trauma

People with addiction problems are often dealing with a lot of past physical, emotional, or sexual traumas. Having endured some form of physical or sexual abuse, which is especially common in women, significantly increases the risk for substance abuse. In many cases, people who have suffered abuse use alcohol, drugs, food, or other unhealthy behaviors to suppress negative emotions. Dealing with past traumas is essential to the healing process.

Upbringing

Being raised in a chaotic environment without a lot of affection and nurturing damages your psychological well-being. These early hurts can be long-lasting and can influence your behavior into adulthood. Having demanding parents who put excessive pressure on you to succeed can also be harmful to your psyche. Trying to live up to someone else's lofty expectations, even your own, can create an enormous amount of stress.

Self Image and Outlook on Life

The way you view yourself and your body can seriously impact your risk for addiction. People with a negative self-image are far more inclined to engage in unhealthy behaviors. If you hate the way you look or feel like you are a failure, then you may feel like it doesn't matter whether or not you take care of yourself or that you don't deserve to treat yourself and your body with the respect and care it needs. Similarly, if you feel like you have no control over your life or that there is no hope for a brighter future, then you are more likely to go down the wrong path. You may turn to unhealthy behaviors to suppress the negative emotions you have about yourself and your life.

Past Successes and Failures

People who see their lives as littered with perceived failures have a tendency to use food, alcohol, drugs, or other behaviors to deal with this negative view. Focusing on your successes—at school, in relationships, in sports, or at work—can mitigate any failures and help keep you from feeling the need to overindulge.

Dealing with Grief

When a loved one dies or when a significant other breaks up with you, it can be emotionally devastating. But why are some people able to bounce back quickly and resume their daily lives while others get mired in their grief and feel like they can't go on? It is likely due to a concept called *brain reserve*. Brain reserve is the cushion of healthy brain function we have to deal with stressful events. The more reserve you have, the better you can cope with the unexpected. The less you have, the harder it is for you to handle tough times and injuries, and the more likely you are to smoke, swig alcohol, or chow down on an entire bag of chocolate-covered pretzels as a coping mechanism. You will learn more about brain reserve in Chapter 9: Boost Your Brain to Get Control.

Social Factors That Make You More Vulnerable to Addiction

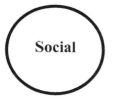

From a *social* perspective it is important to look at the stresses in your life, including relationships, work, school, and finances. There are many life events and stresses that can trigger the inclination to develop bad habits. Often they result from some sort of relationship difficulty or loss, such as a breakup or divorce. Financial troubles can also eat away at you. Overwhelming responsibilities at work and home can make you want to find a way to escape from daily stresses. Even your daily habits and hobbies can alter your brain chemistry and make you more prone to addiction. In most cases, it is when a number of stresses start piling on at the same time that you become more prone to addiction.

Relationships

Your relationships with your parents, grandparents, siblings, children, significant other, friends, and coworkers are so important to your health and well-being. In today's mobile society, however, it can be difficult to develop meaningful relationships. Many people move away from their hometown to find work, commute long hours from home to work, or move around a lot, making it harder to forge lasting friendships and strong family ties. The high rate of divorce in our society also splits up families and abruptly severs friendships.

A lack of social connections causes negative changes in the brain that can lead to trouble in your life. The quality of the relationships in your life is just as important as the quantity. Difficult relationships that are a source of stress, anger, and negative emotions are damaging to the brain. Many people with addictions have troubled relationships with the people in their lives or have few social connections.

Brianna, sixteen, played on her school's volleyball team and counted her teammates as her best friends. They did everything together—going to the movies, shopping at the mall, listening to music, and just hanging out. But all that changed when her teammates found out that Brianna had gotten drunk at a party and had sex with one of the girl's boyfriends. Brianna got kicked off the squad and the team shunned her. Brianna's entire social circle evaporated, and she was unbearably lonely. Desperate for friendships, she started hanging out with the "losers" and adopting their bad behaviors, which included drinking and doing drugs. Granted, Brianna's bad judgment while drunk initiated her expulsion from the group, but the social isolation drove her deeper into addiction.

Even if your life is filled with people you love, you can still experience a lot of stress from your relationships. If your wife is fighting cancer, your daughter has decided to drop out of high school, or your father has been diagnosed with Alzheimer's disease, it can affect your life too. We are social beings and the health and happiness of our loved ones directly impact our own sense of well-being.

Work and School

Mean bosses, rude customers, backstabbing coworkers—the people at work can make your life miserable. Having a demanding workload or performing a job you hate can also add to the stress in your life. Similarly, problems with classmates or teachers at school can cause problems with self-image and confidence. Trying to "do it all" at work, at school, at home, at church, and in your relationships can sap your energy and leave you feeling frazzled.

If you feel overwhelmed by your obligations, you may be inclined to take drugs that enhance performance. This has become an increasing problem on college campuses nationwide. A fascinating article in a 2009 issue of *The New Yorker* detailed the growing use of "neuroenhancers," drugs that young people believe will help them do it all: get better grades, work longer hours, stay up late partying with friends, and more. In the medical literature, statistics about the off-label usage of prescription stimulants on college campuses vary from about 7 percent up to almost 35 percent of the student body. In one survey of 390 college students in the *Journal of Attention Disorder*, 60 percent of those surveyed reported knowing students who misused prescription stimulants and 50 percent said that the drugs were easy to get on campus. A 2006 study involving 4,580 college students found that among those who had used prescription stimulants for off-label purposes, the most common reasons were to help with concentration, studying, and alertness.

Finances

Financial problems can be a tremendous source of stress, and many people blame money woes for their addictions. Often, people suffering from economic hardships turn to substances and behaviors that temporarily help them forget their troubles. Unfortunately, many of the things people do in an attempt to escape from their problems end up worsening their financial situation. The cost of buying alcohol, drugs, or even cigarettes or snack foods adds up fast. People with addictions tend to miss more days of work and get fewer promotions, which lowers their income potential.

Thrilling Behavior

In his intriguing book *Thrilled to Death: How the Endless Pursuit of Pleasure Is Leaving Us Numb*, psychologist Archibald Hart warns that text messaging, email, video games, and television can overstimulate our pleasure centers in the same way cocaine does. We all know people who are so glued to their BlackBerry that they call it a "CrackBerry." For these people, every time their mobile device pings to signal a new incoming message, it causes a release of dopamine in the brain. With video gamers, dopamine is being released constantly throughout the game. And with television, the quick-cut, high-intensity action is overstimulating.

These technologies are effectively wearing out our pleasure centers. In effect, our fast-paced, pleasure-seeking lifestyle is robbing us of the ability to experience joy from the simple things in life. Things that used to make us feel happy leave us feeling numb. Hart goes on to suggest that our excessive pursuit of constant thrills may contribute to emotional problems, such as depression and anxiety, as well as addictions to drugs, alcohol, Internet gambling, pornography, or compulsive shopping.

Spiritual Factors That Make You More Vulnerable to Addiction

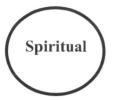

From a *spiritual* standpoint, it is critical to look at what your life means and if you have a sense of purpose or a connection to something greater than yourself. Spiritual factors also tie in to your core values and sense of morality—what is right and wrong in your eyes. If you don't feel like your life matters, you are less inclined to take good care of yourself. Similarly, if you don't feel connected to something larger than yourself, you may not feel accountable for your actions. After all, if you don't believe that you are accountable for your actions, then why should you do the right thing?

Let's look at how spiritual factors played into addiction for Jake, the entrepreneur mentioned in the introduction to this chapter. He felt absolutely no connection to anything other than himself and had no purpose in his life other than making money. Although he was very good at building his financial empire, it didn't bring him the satisfaction he thought it would. This was part of the problem that led him to abuse cocaine and alcohol. As part of the healing process, he became a philanthropist and joined the boards of several charities that help people with substance abuse problems. This made him feel like he was doing something important with his life, something that mattered, and it filled him with a sense of purpose that has helped him stay away from drugs and alcohol.

The Road to Healing

In order to heal, you need to address all four pillars. If you discover that you have ADD and treat it but don't deal with the negative self-image you developed due to doing poorly in school (likely due to your ADD), you will never get completely well. By getting on a brain healthy program, taking care of any brain problems, dealing with your emotional issues, developing a strong social support system, minimizing the stresses in your daily life, and developing a sense of purpose and meaning in your life, you can get on the road to recovery.

In this book we use this comprehensive bio-psycho-social-spiritual approach to help you heal and ultimately thrive. In Part Two you will discover the ten steps to unchain your brain so you can break free from your addictions.

1. Know your motivation (spiritual healing)

2. Get the right evaluation (biological, psychological, social, and spiritual healing)

3. Know your brain type (biological healing)

4. Boost your brain to get control (biological healing)

5. Craving control (biological, psychological, and social healing)

6. Eat right to think right and heal from your addiction (biological healing)

7. Kill the Addiction ANTs that infest your brain and keep you in chains (psychological healing)

8. Manage your stress that triggers relapse (psychological and social healing)

9. H-A-L-T plus: overcome the barriers that keep you from conquering your addictions (biological, psychological, and social healing)

10. Get well, beyond yourself (social and spiritual healing)

UNCHAIN YOUR BRAIN CHECKLIST

- ✓ Know the biological contributors to addiction.

- ✓ Know the psychological contributors to addiction.

- ✓ Know the social contributors to addiction.

- ✓ Know the spiritual contributors to addiction.

- ✓ Heal any biological problems.

- ✓ Heal any psychological problems.

- ✓ Heal any social problems.

- ✓ Heal any spiritual problems.

Part Two

10 STEPS TO BREAKING FREE FROM THE ADDICTIONS THAT STEAL YOUR LIFE

Chapter 6

Step #1

KNOW YOUR MOTIVATION

To Drive Your Desire to Change

It sometimes seems that intense desire creates not only its own opportunities, but its own talents. – Eric Hoffer

My co-author David was attending a medical conference in Chicago in 1989 when he got a frantic call from Bill Graham, the legendary rock concert promoter. Graham was on tour with the Grateful Dead and told David, "Jerry Garcia is strung out, and you have to do something." David headed to the band's hotel, where he had to snake his way through a sea of tie-dye-clad groupies and billows of marijuana smoke to get to Garcia's room. Inside, he found Graham and Garcia's band mates, bass player Phil Lesh and rhythm guitarist Bob Weir, who was in recovery from hard drugs.

Drugs and rock'n'roll had been a way of life for Garcia for decades. While on tour with The Dead, people would give him all the drugs he wanted. He would often smoke heroin backstage just to make himself feel better. The years of hard partying and touring had not been kind to Garcia. He was severely overweight, he had diabetes, and he had even slipped into a diabetic coma a few years earlier. But that wasn't enough to make him want to change his ways.

The band told Garcia that he was killing himself with drugs, and they were staging an intervention. It wasn't the first intervention they had tried. Garcia had run away from the last one and subsequently gotten arrested for possession. This time, though, his band mates told him that they would no longer go out on the road with him unless he got help for his addiction. For Garcia, touring with the band and playing music for thousands of people was what he loved most in life. The threat of losing that is what finally motivated him to change and enter a holistic addiction treatment center.

For most people, it takes something drastic to inspire change. Jenna, thirty-six, was no different. She had been a binge eater since she was a teenager. Her nighttime binges usually started innocently enough with a scoop of butter pecan ice cream. But by the end of the evening, she would have polished off the entire half-gallon container of ice cream, eaten a whole bag of chocolate chip cookies, downed several king-sized candy bars, and stuffed herself with a plate of brownies. Her binges could add up to as many as ten thousand calories in a single sitting.

The extra calories had added up and she now tipped the scales at 315 pounds on her five-foot-four-inch frame. She also had type 2 diabetes, high cholesterol, high triglycerides, sleep apnea that raised her risk for Alzheimer's disease, and itchy rashes on her thighs from the constant chafing. But that wasn't enough to motivate her to want to change.

It wasn't until Jenna found out that she was pregnant with a baby girl that it really hit her. If she wanted to survive long enough to see her unborn child grow up into adulthood she would have to change her ways. She was also terrified that she would be a bad role model and that her daughter would end up being fat too, and she didn't want her little girl to have to endure the humiliation and self-loathing she lived with every day.

The tiny life that was growing inside her motivated Jenna to want to be healthy. That's when Jenna finally sought professional help for her binge eating, tossed the junk food in the trash, started an exercise program, and began taking care of herself.

In order for you to break free from the chains of addiction, you must know your motivation. Is it to:

- get healthy?
- live long?
- have great relationships?
- be smarter?
- look younger?
- have a better brain?
- have more money?
- keep your spouse from divorcing you?
- prevent another potentially fatal overdose?
- avoid flunking out of college?
- reverse diabetes, lung cancer, or other health risks?
- stop beating yourself up about your weight, drinking, or gambling?
- stop getting arrested or going to jail?
- avoid getting fired?
- avoid losing your home and living on the streets?

Truth and Consequences: The First Step to Change is Pain

It isn't easy to change, which is why most of us are so reluctant to do it. Our brains get comfortable with our daily habits and patterns, even if they are unhealthy for us. In order to change our habits, the brain has to be rewired and develop a whole new system, and it fights that process.

That's why even though you know that it would be better for you to stop overeating, smoking, or drinking alcohol, you don't do it. It is only when those habits cause enough pain in your life that you finally make the decision to change, like Jenna who couldn't bear the thought of seeing her little girl turn out like her.

You know how powerful pain can be. On a day when you feel fine, there is no way you would spend $8 for a bottle of one hundred aspirin, but if you have a headache, you would gladly fork over $20 for a single one. It's the same with your addictions. Until you are consumed with pain and your life becomes unmanageable, you will continue to let your addictions control you, unless your brain works right and you kick in enough forethought.

It took a lot more than just one thing to cause enough pain to make twenty-eight-year-old Kimo want to quit smoking methamphetamine. It took getting his teeth knocked out in a fight over meth, having his wife threaten to divorce him, AND getting arrested before he realized that he needed help to battle his addiction.

For Maxine, fifty-seven, it was the need for a liver transplant due to decades of drinking. When she discovered that alcoholics have to be in recovery for six month to be eligible for a liver transplant, she knew she had to change...OR DIE. That is the ultimate consequence.

I receive many emails and letters from people who have heard about my work and are terrified of what their brain will look like. They are so sure they have caused a lot of damage due to their drinking or drug use that it motivates them to stop using. Brain imaging is so powerful.

The pain and consequences that inspire change are different for each person. In your case, it might be financial problems, relationship woes, legal troubles, or health conditions. In order for you to change, you need to understand why you are uncomfortable. Only then can you make the decision to change your brain so you can break free from your addictions.

What are the consequences that have brought you or your loved one to this juncture? Write them down here or use a separate sheet of paper. Don't leave anything out no matter how trivial you may believe it to be. When you have your list, mark the consequences that matter most to you, that brought you the most shame, or that you want to make sure you never experience again.

Consequences of My Addiction

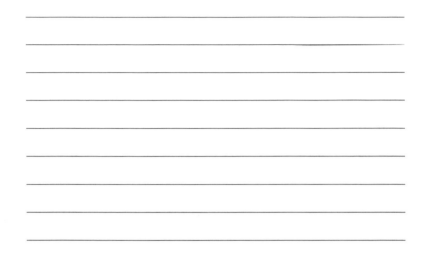

Hope: You've Got to Have It

Unless you have hope, you are never going to make the decision to change. Hope is what makes you believe that you can change and that your life will be better if you succeed in changing your ways.

How do you find that hope? Sometimes it can be generated by someone you respect—a teacher, a pastor, a doctor, or an author. Our great hope is that this book will infuse you with hope so you will follow the ten steps to break free from your addictions. We have seen it work for so many people, and it can work for you.

For seventeen-year-old Kasey, hope wasn't easy to come by. She was kicked out of one treatment center because she told them she didn't want to be there because she didn't think she needed help and didn't think they could make her change. After a subsequent stint in juvenile hall and the threat of being institutionalized, Kasey finally came to the conclusion that she did need help after all. But all the treatment facilities her parents contacted turned her down based on her experience at that first center. This made her feel even more hopeless.

Finally, her parents found a treatment center—one that specialized in treating teenage girls—that would accept her. There, Kasey found counselors who truly cared about her and believed in her ability to change. It was their belief in her that gave her hope and the willingness to work with them instead of against them. Filled with that hope, Kasey overcame her addictions and is happy with her life for the first time in years.

What are the things that inspire a feeling of hope for you? Create a list of people, books, songs, and anything else that makes you feel hopeful about your ability to change.

My Hope List

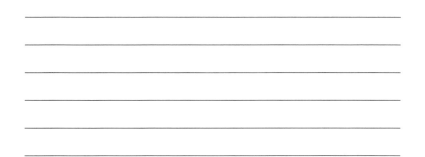

What Does Your Life Mean and Why Do You Care?

In order to stay motivated to change, you need to know why your life is important. For me, I have an amazing wife, four wonderful children, and a new grandson, Elias. My grandfather was one of the most important people in my whole life. I was named after him, and he was my best friend growing up. I know how important grandparents can be. The day Elias was born I thought about my grandfather all day long. I want to be healthy to be able to love Elias like my grandfather loved me.

When I think about what's really important to me, no amount of pizza, doughnuts, or double fudge chocolate chip brownies is worth the price of damaging my health and stealing the time I have with my family. You have to focus on your motivation, or food, cigarettes, drugs, or whatever it is that tempts you will control you. Scientists have found that the doughnuts, double fudge chocolate chip cookies, cigarettes, video games, and cocaine all work on the dopamine centers of the brain and can be totally addictive.

Like me, David has a wonderful family—a wife who is dedicated to recovery, four loving children, and three adorable grandchildren. They are what keep him motivated to stay clean and sober and to be as healthy as he can possibly be. When he is eating brain healthy foods, exercising on his stair climber, or playing basketball, he is thinking about how he is improving his health so he can be around longer to love his grandchildren. The lure of pot, LSD, and alcohol just isn't as strong as his desire to be a loving and caring husband, father, and grandfather.

So, what motivates you to change? Is it health or is it fear? Some people, me included, require fear.

I finally lost the extra twenty pounds I had been carrying around because I kept reading studies like the one from the University of Pittsburgh where researchers found that the brains of overweight people looked eight to sixteen years older than healthy people. Given that your brain controls everything you do, including how much love you have in your life and how much money you make, you do not want a smaller brain! Considering my line of work, having a smaller brain is not an option.

If your motivation is like mine or like David's and it involves the people you love, put up their pictures where you can see them every day. This is my screensaver.

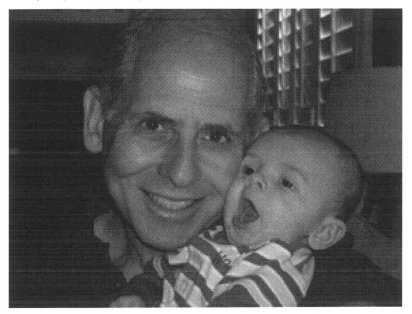

David also keeps pictures of his grandchildren where he can look at them every day. Here are a few of his favorites.

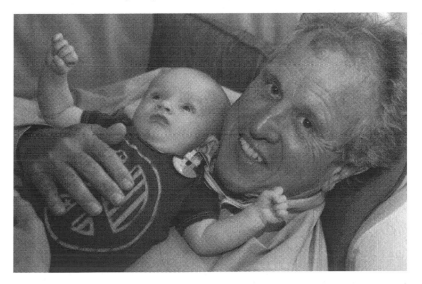

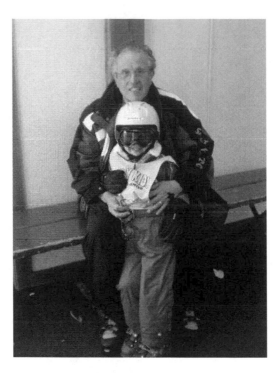

So, what is your specific motivation to change? Write it down and put it where you can see it every day. Be positive:

"I want to live long."

"I want to have great energy."

"I want to look great."

"I want to be smart."

"I want to have better relationships."

My Motivation to Change

_____

_____

_____

_____

_____

_____

Find Your Bliss

One of the keys to staying motivated is finding your bliss—
something you can be passionate about that keeps you feeling
energized and excited. Of course, this does NOT mean something
addictive. Many people mistake an addiction to food, sex, or wine
for passion. You have to be careful not to get too much pleasure
from your passions, or your reward system could hijack your brain.

For David and me, our passion is helping people improve their
brain health so they can have better lives, stronger relationships,
more successful careers, healthier bodies, and more happiness.
With each patient success story, we are rewarded with a healthy
dose of dopamine that makes us want to continue reproducing that
success.

You need to fall in love with something other than your
addiction, something that serves you. First, you need to fall in love
with your own brain. I'll talk more about this in Chapter 9: Boost
Your Brain to Get Control.

For Kendra, thirty-one, it took a long time to find her bliss. In
high school, she developed bulimia. Her weight had begun to creep
up, and she started making herself throw up in an effort to avoid
getting fat. She would binge on pizza, bacon cheeseburgers, and
lasagna and then feel so guilty about it that she would head to the
bathroom to purge. This unhealthy relationship with food
continued for a decade before she finally sought help.

In treatment, Kendra was encouraged to help out in the organic
garden at the treatment facility. By planting, nurturing, and eating

the healthy vegetables and fruits from the garden, her relationship with food slowly began to change. The feelings of guilt and revulsion that she had so long associated with food and eating began to dissipate. Instead, she began to realize that putting nutritious foods in her body made her feel good and helped her maintain a healthy weight.

Kendra eventually fell in love with organic gardening and cooking. She was amazed by the difference in her life—her overall health, energy levels, and moods vastly improved—that she wanted to share her newly gained knowledge with others. That's when she launched an organic foods catering business. Her work makes her feel like she is doing something important with her life and that helps keep her from falling into her old destructive behaviors.

I urge you to find your bliss. What are the things you are passionate about? Music? Cooking? Sports (without head injury risk, of course)? Writing? Fashion? Animals? Your kids? Get a piece of paper and write down all the things you love or that make you happy. If you are in the clutches of addiction, you may not feel like there is anything you care about other than your addiction. Don't get discouraged. Give yourself some time. You may not discover your true passion until your brain starts to heal.

My Bliss List

_____

_____

_____

_____

_____

_____

Get in Touch With Your Spiritual Side

People who have a serious addiction problem must have a spiritual program. This doesn't necessarily mean organized religion, although that can be very beneficial for some people. Think of spirituality in the broader sense of feeling connected to something greater than yourself, feeling connected to the earth, feeling connected to past generations, and feeling connected to future generations. Having a sense of belonging is an important step in the healing process.

Developing a sense of accountability for your actions also promotes healing. When you feel like you are accountable to no one, who cares if you smash up your car, lose your job, or create havoc in your relationships? When you feel accountable to a higher power or to your own moral compass, then your actions matter and it becomes important to do the right thing.

This leads you to define your own sense of morality and to clarify your values. What is important to you? How do you want to treat people? How do you want to treat yourself? How do you want to behave in society? Do you want to lie, cheat, and steal to fuel your addiction, or do you want to be honest, loving, and forgiving? Including some form of spirituality is critical to helping you overcome your addictions.

Many treatment programs, such as Alcoholics Anonymous, have a spiritual component. Here are a few examples of others that focus on spirituality and a look at why they can be successful.

I was eighteen years old when I volunteered to work with Teen Challenge, a faith-based treatment program for young people with substance abuse problems. Teen Challenge has an impressive track record. After being a neuroscientist for decades now, I have discovered why it works so well. There are three specific "brain-centered" reasons why the program is successful. It is because they provide the three Fs: frontal lobes, family (limbic bonding), and fear.

Frontal lobes (rules). As we have seen, the front part of your brain, the prefrontal cortex, is involved with executive functions, such as rule-oriented behavior, morals, and internal supervision. It is the little voice in your head that helps you decide between right and wrong. Teen Challenge introduces its clients to the New Testament, which contains a very clear set of guidelines and rules. It gives its students structure. I often say it gives people an extra frontal lobe to help supervise their lives.

Family (limbic bonding). People who are addicts often do not feel a connection to anything or anyone. They are often estranged from their families and shunned by their former friends because of their erratic and irresponsible behavior. But the human brain needs bonding in order to achieve optimal functioning. At Teen Challenge the counselors, other patients, and the church group take on the role of a family support group. This feeds the limbic area of the brain, which is involved in motivation and mood control.

Fear and anxiety (what you do has consequences). Studies show that impulsive addicts have low levels of anxiety. In response to stress, they actually have lower sweat gland activity and lower heart rates than non-addicts, which means they don't feel nervous about doing risky things. The Teen Challenge program, however, introduces addicts to the concept of Hell, and they are not kidding. It teaches that if you're not right with God, then you will go to Hell for eternity. That can strike fear in even the most hard-core substance abusers. And, if Hell is a concept that is too far off for you to have impact, they teach you about the Rapture, that Jesus may come back tomorrow, and if you are not ready, you will be left behind. For many, that gets their attention. "Are you ready?" This is not religion light—they are serious!

Anxiety mixed with frontal lobe help and limbic bonding
is the perfect combination for people with addictions.

Here is another example of a faith-based treatment program that boasts a high success rate. One media story reported that 93 percent of the people who participate in this program never use drugs again. Communita Cenacolo America, which was founded by Sister Elvira Petrozzi in Italy, claims it is not a therapeutic program but rather a "School of Life." The program is largely based on prayer and requires daily recitation of the Rosary, which involves repeated sequences of specific prayers. Another daily requirement is physical work, such as construction, carpentry, cooking, and gardening.

Like Teen Challenge, this program offers frontal lobes (rules and structured daily life) and family. In place of the fear, however, is facing the truth about themselves, being forgiving, and finally looking beyond themselves to volunteer to help others. Learning to give back to your family, community, and planet can be very important in keeping you motivated to stay on track.

Remember that the concept of spirituality doesn't apply only to religion. It also involves stepping outside of yourself to think about and help others. Getting involved in your community is an ideal way to develop a sense of purpose and a feeling that you are doing something important. You will likely find that doing good for others does you a lot of good, too. Do a quick Internet search to find opportunities to volunteer in your area.

One-Page Miracle

One of the most powerful yet simple exercises I have designed is called the One-Page Miracle. It will help guide nearly all of your thoughts words, and actions. It is called the One-Page "Miracle" because I've seen this exercise quickly focus and change many people's lives. It is particularly effective for people with addictions because it makes you focus on what is truly important to you and forces you to think about long-term goals rather than just the immediate gratification that comes from addictive substances and behaviors. As you will see, it is an all-encompassing bio-psycho-social-spiritual exercise that includes your hopes and dreams for all of these areas.

Directions: Either make copies of the following "My One-Page Miracle" or take a sheet of paper and clearly write out a rough draft of your major goals for the four pillars of healing: biological, psychological, social, and spiritual. If you are using a piece of paper, include "brain health," "physical health," and "cravings" under "Biological." Under "Psychological," write "emotional health," and "thinking patterns." Under "Social," include "spouse," "children," "extended family/friends," "work/school," and "money." Under "Spiritual," write "spirituality," "character," "passions," and "community."

Next to each subheading succinctly write out what's important to you in that area. Write what you want, not what you don't want. Be positive and use the first person. Write what you want with confidence and the expectation that you will make it happen. Keep the paper with you so that you can work on it over several days or weeks.

After you finish with the initial draft (you'll want to update it frequently), place this piece of paper where you can see it every day, such as on your refrigerator, by your bedside, or on the bathroom mirror. In that way, every day you focus your eyes on what's important to you. This makes it easier to match your behavior to what you want. Your life becomes more conscious and you spend your energy on goals that are important to you.

Here is an example I did with one of my patients who came to see me at the insistence of his wife after he started abusing alcohol, gambled away their savings, developed wild mood swings, and was nearly fired from his job due to his erratic behavior. Nicholas was estranged from his family and shunned by several of his friends because he borrowed money from them and then lost it gambling. Nicholas works as a computer programmer for a major corporation, but he had always dreamed of doing something more artistic. He is married with one child. Nicholas' brain SPECT scans showed that he had suffered a head injury, and it was after experiencing the brain trauma that he developed significant impulse control problems, addiction, and mood swings. In therapy, Nicholas also revealed that his father had been verbally and physically abusive.

After you look at the example on the following page, fill out the OPM for yourself. If you have prefrontal cortex challenges, which are common in people with addictions, this exercise will be very helpful for you. After you complete this exercise, put it up where you can see and read it every day. It is a great idea to start off each day by reading your OPM to get focused on what really matters to you. Then before you do or say something, ask yourself if your potential behavior fits your goals.

NICHOLAS' ONE-PAGE MIRACLE
What Do I Want? What Am I Doing To Make It Happen?

BIOLOGICAL—to be the healthiest I can be

Brain health: To love my brain, protect it from toxins like alcohol, and engage in new learning.

Physical health: To take care of my body on a daily basis, exercise, eat well, and get good sleep.

Cravings: To do what's necessary to control my cravings for alcohol and my compulsion to gamble.

PSYCHOLOGICAL—to love, respect, and be forgiving of myself

Emotional health: To deal with past emotional traumas and to get my moods under control.

Thinking patterns: To kill the ANTs (automatic negative thoughts) with my ANTeater, to focus on the positive, and to be grateful every day.

SOCIAL—to be connected to those I love and to develop a strong support group

Spouse: To create a close, kind, caring, loving partnership with my wife. I want her to know how much I care about her. I want to act in a way that makes her feel less worried about me.

Children: To be a firm, kind, positive, predictable presence in my child's life. I want to be a good role model so I can help her to develop into a happy, responsible person.

Extended family/friends: To reconnect with my parents, siblings, and friends and to show them I am deserving of their trust.

Work/school: To be a reliable employee so I can be successful.

Money: To be a good steward and wise spender.

SPIRITUAL—to feel connected to a higher power

Spirituality: To attend group meetings regularly, attend church regularly, and pray and meditate daily.

Character: To be honest, thoughtful, kind, and trustworthy. To live with integrity.

Passions: To pursue my love for drawing by taking an evening art class.

Community: To volunteer for a local children's charity.

MY ONE-PAGE MIRACLE
What Do I Want? What Am I Doing To Make It Happen?

BIOLOGICAL

Brain
Health: _____

Physical: _____

Health: _____

Cravings: _____

_____

PSYCHOLOGICAL

Emotional _____

Health: _____

Thinking _____

Patterns: _____

SOCIAL

Spouse: _____

_____

Children: _____

_____

Family/ _____

Friends: _____

Work/ _____

School: _____

Money: _____

_____

SPIRITUAL

Spirituality: _____

_____

Character: _____

_____

Passions: _____

_____

Community: _____

_____

UNCHAIN YOUR BRAIN CHECKLIST

✓ Take stock of the consequences of your addiction.

✓ Look at your Hope List and read, watch, or listen to the things that inspire you on a daily basis and whenever you feel discouraged or hopeless.

✓ Write down the specific things that are motivating you to change.

✓ Find something other than your addiction that you can be passionate about.

✓ Focus on the reasons why you must be healthy every day, or the doughnuts, cigarettes, drugs, or alcohol will always win.

✓ Develop a sense of being connected with a higher power, the earth, and other people.

✓ Look at your One-Page Miracle every day and focus on your goals.

Chapter 7

Step #2

GET THE RIGHT EVALUATION

A Bio-Psycho-Social-Spiritual Approach
Get a clear picture of what is going on in your brain,
body, and life.

When Jacob was thirty-four, he and his wife were in a car accident that took her life and left him with a serious concussion. Now a grief-stricken single father with a rambunctious four-year-old, he couldn't cope with the stress. When a woman he had just started dating suggested they smoke methamphetamine because it would make sex better, he said, "Okay." This was completely out of character for Jacob, who had smoked pot a few times in high school and college, but had never tried hard drugs before. His new girlfriend was right about the meth. They had mind-blowing sex. Whenever she came over, they would smoke meth before having sex. Then Jacob couldn't wait until their weekend date, and he started smoking it at least once a day.

One day, as he lit the meth, he dropped his lighter on the floor and burned his house down. He and his son were both rushed to the hospital with severe burns. Jacob ended up losing his son to foster care and went to jail. When he got out, he was forced into treatment. In treatment, the evaluation included a detailed family history, addressing his grief and stress issues, and examining environmental triggers like his girlfriend who encouraged him to smoke meth. In spite of all the help he received through treatment, Jacob couldn't resist the lure of meth and started smoking it again.

What was missing from his evaluation? When Jacob landed in David's care, David ordered a brain scan from us and discovered

117

that Jacob had suffered severe brain trauma, probably from the car accident that had killed his wife. The damage to his brain was making him more impulsive and reckless. When Jacob started the treatment we recommended, his brain health improved and with all the other support offered in treatment, he was able to stay clean.

Jacob's Brain Before Treatment

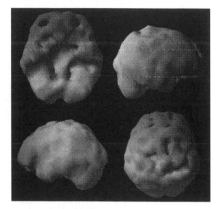

Jacob's Brain After Treatment

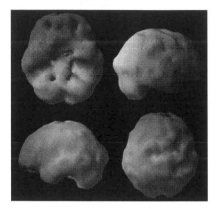

Leona, a fifty-one-year-old single mother of two teenagers, always felt fatigued and could barely make it through the day without falling asleep at her desk at work. One day, she decided to try her son's Ritalin (a prescription stimulant used to treat ADD)—it worked for her son and helped him get more accomplished during the day so maybe it would help her too. Soon, she was taking it every day and often felt so fidgety at night that she would have a few drinks to help her calm down and sleep.

Eventually, she recognized that she had a problem and wanted to get it treated so she went to her doctor, who recommended she join a support group. Leona faithfully attended meetings, where they discussed the many psychological and social reasons that contributed to her drug use and drinking. She tried really hard to abstain from taking the Ritalin, but she felt so lethargic she just couldn't quit.

What was missing from her evaluation that could have helped

her be more successful with treatment? Nobody thought to check Leona's physical health and hormone levels. A simple blood test showed that Leona's thyroid levels were very low, which can cause excessive fatigue and sluggishness. When she balanced her thyroid, she felt more energetic and didn't feel the need for the stimulant.

Kylia was thirteen years old when her nineteen-year-old cousin raped her. She was so humiliated she never told her parents what happened. Ever since the terrible incident, she felt tense and nervous, as if she was always waiting for something bad to happen. A few years later, she found some painkillers in her parents' medicine cabinet and decided to take them to help her calm down. She liked the way they took the edge off and got hooked. She also started sleeping around with a lot of the guys at school. When her parents walked in on her having scx in their bedroom and found out about her drug habit, they shipped her off to a boarding school for problem kids that did regular urine screenings for drugs. Kylia failed the tests repeatedly and got kicked out of the school.

What was missing from her evaluation? Nobody ever addressed the psychological trauma Kylia had experienced so she never dealt with it head on. She was unable to let go of the hurt and shame she felt, which played into her addiction. On brain imaging we have seen a very specific pattern for patients with posttraumatic stress disorder. We call it the "diamond plus" pattern, where there is too much activity in the anterior cingulate gyrus (the brain's gear shifter gets stuck on negative thoughts or traumatic events), the basal ganglia (increased anxiety), deep limbic system (sadness), and right outside temporal lobe (processing the intentions of others).

Posttraumatic Stress Disorder—Diamond Plus Pattern

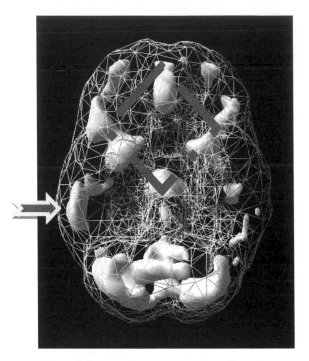

Top of diamond—anterior cingulate (gets stuck)
Sides of diamond—basal ganglia (anxiety)
Bottom of diamond—deep limbic (sadness)
Arrow—right lateral temporal lobe (processing
intention of others, watching for something bad to
happen)

One of the most exciting studies I have published with my colleagues is on posttraumatic stress disorder where we demonstrated that with a specific treatment called EMDR (eye movement desensitization and reprocessing) the brain can change, and the diamond plus pattern settles down.

Jarrell, thirty-three, worked in the marketing department at an Internet company and had to juggle numerous projects at the same time. He couldn't keep it all organized and struggled to get his work done on time. Worried he might get fired, Jarrell started doing cocaine to help him stay up at night to finish his work. He would get such a buzz that he would have to take prescription sleeping pills on the weekends to get any rest. That's when Jarrell's company implemented a new drug screening program and made all current employees submit to a drug test. When Jarrell's test came up positive, he was fired on the spot. That's what forced him into treatment. Jarrell tried to follow the program but he just couldn't do it. He was either late for the meetings or forgot to go and never got around to doing the self-help work or reading the materials they gave him.

What was missing from his evaluation? Nobody thought to examine if there was a biological reason why Jarrell was having so much trouble at work. At the Amen Clinics, we discovered he had ADD, which makes it hard to focus, stay organized, and meet deadlines. On the proper medication, Jarrell was able to stay focused on his recovery.

Getting a comprehensive evaluation is critical to healing. Make sure you seek out an addiction professional, treatment program, or support group that examines all four pillars and how they are involved in your problem. In this chapter, I will share our approach so you can have a blueprint of what your evaluation should include.

Biological Evaluations

At the Amen Clinics, we take a complete look at the health of the brain and body when treating patients with addictions. Typically, this involves evaluating the health of your brain using SPECT imaging, checking your important health numbers, and taking a detailed family history.

1. Know your brain.

In our clinics, we use SPECT brain imaging to evaluate the health of your brain and detect brain dysfunction. Getting a clear picture of your brain health can help identify brain problems, such as abnormal blood flow, head injuries, ADD, depression, anxiety, or dementia, which can increase your risk for addiction and relapse.

For many years, I have known that not everyone is able to get a brain scan to check on the health of his or her brain. So, in order to bring the life-changing information I have learned through my imaging work to the most people, I have developed a series of questionnaires to help predict the areas of strengths and vulnerabilities of the brain. You can take the Unchain Your Brain Master Questionnaire in Appendix A or take an expanded version online to get an idea of the health of your brain. Also check Chapter 8: Know Your Brain Type to learn more about the six types of addicts, which type you are, and how knowing this information can help you break free from addiction.

Is there abnormal blood flow in the brain? The SPECT brain scans show blood flow activity in the brain, indicating areas that are working well, areas that are not working hard enough, and areas that are working too hard.

When blood flow levels are low, it can reduce impulse control and lower overall brain activity, which makes you more likely to do stupid things. When brains don't work hard enough, people tend to use substances like cocaine or thrilling behaviors to stimulate the brain. A 2010 brain SPECT imaging study from Brazil found that low cerebral blood flow is common in adolescents who are dependent on multiple drugs. The team of researchers discovered that the younger the drug user, the more areas of low blood flow in the brain. Many factors cause low blood flow to the brain.

Causes of Low Blood Flow to the Brain

- Genetics
- Brain injuries
- Toxicity
- Alcohol
- Drug abuse
- Environmental toxins

- Lack of oxygen (near-drowning incidents, for example)
- Exposure to mold
- Sleep apnea
- Chronic lack of sleep
- Vascular disease
- Diabetes
- Many medications
- Lack of nutrients
- Low blood sugar
- Dehydration
- Low thyroid levels
- Imbalanced hormones
- Smoking and secondhand smoke
- Prior brain infection
- Anemia
- Food allergies

When blood flow levels are too high, brains work too hard and people have a tendency for obsessive thoughts or compulsive behaviors. People with obsessive-compulsive disorder, many anxiety disorders, posttraumatic stress disorder, and anorexia typically have overactive brains. When you have an overactive brain, you are more likely to use substances like alcohol, downers, and simple carbohydrates to calm your brain. Increased brain activity can be the result of a wide number of issues.

Causes of Too Much Brain Activity

- Genetics
- Past emotional trauma
- Posttraumatic stress disorder
- PMS
- Allergies
- Autoimmune disorders, initially
- Inflammation
- Acute stress
- Grief

- Food allergies
- Excessive electrical activity in the brain

Have you ever had a head injury? After looking at more than 57,000 brain scans, it has become clear to me that even mild physical trauma can damage the brain and increase your risk for addiction. Alcoholism, drug abuse, and eating disorders are all more common in people who have experienced head injuries. In a 2007 study analyzing data from 7,784 adults in state-funded substance abuse treatment, researchers found that nearly one-third of them had experienced a traumatic brain injury with loss of consciousness.

This is a huge concern considering the staggering number of soldiers returning from Iraq and Afghanistan with traumatic brain injuries. According to statistics traumatic brain injury is the most common war wound suffered, affecting 15 percent of these returning soldiers. But you don't need to be hit by a roadside bomb or even lose consciousness for a brain injury to increase your risk for out-of-control behavior. Falling off your bunk bed as a child, tripping down a flight of stairs, playing contact sports like football, or having a bicycle accident can harm your brain and make you more vulnerable to the grips of addiction.

Several years ago, I wrote an article about how head trauma can change everything in your life. The day the paper hit the newsstands, I got a call from a distraught mom who said she had to see me immediately. Later that night at the Amen Clinics, she explained that her son, Marcus, had gotten into a bike accident at age sixteen. He hit the curb, flew over the handlebars, and landed on his head. He was unconscious for about thirty minutes and suffered what doctors called a "mild" concussion.

Prior to the accident, Marcus had been getting straight As in school and was a good, loving person. That all changed after the accident. His grades dropped, he became mean and surly, and he started drinking alcohol. At age twenty, Marcus shot and killed himself. His mother wept as she related this tragic story. I cried too. She was convinced that she had been a bad mother and that her son's suicide was her fault in some way. Like many parents, she had no clue that a head injury could have such a terrible impact on a person's life. For her son, it proved to be lethal.

Do you have any psychiatric disorders? Having mental health issues, which are actually brain disorders, such as ADD, depression, bipolar disorder, or anxiety disorders can fuel addiction and increase your odds for relapse. People diagnosed with mood or anxiety disorders or antisocial disorders are about twice as likely to have a drug dependency problem and are more likely to smoke cigarettes. Scientific evidence shows that among adolescents seeking treatment for substance abuse, 50-90 percent also suffer from some form of psychiatric disorder.

Children and adults with untreated attention deficit disorder (ADD) or attention deficit hyperactivity disorder (ADHD), which are just different names for the same condition, are also at increased risk for addiction. According to one study, half of all people with ADHD will develop a substance abuse problem if it remains untreated. A 2005 report in the journal *Pediatrics* found that having prior or current ADHD not only doubles your risk of developing a substance abuse problem, but also makes you more prone to become addicted at an earlier age and results in a greater intensity of abuse. Having untreated ADD also gives you a significantly higher chance of being overweight.

Why does having ADD so dramatically raise the risk for addiction? ADD is associated with low activity in the prefrontal cortex, which likely contributes to the brain's reward system going haywire. It increases impulsivity, decreases judgment, reduces attention span, and lowers the ability to focus—all of which make for a powerfully detrimental combination. Low activity in the prefrontal cortex has also been linked to a greater risk for relapse among substance abusers.

It is important to understand, however, that substance abuse can alter your behaviors and mimic the symptoms of mental health disorders. When seventeen-year-old Shannon entered treatment, she had terrible mood swings and appeared to have bipolar disorder. A few weeks later after abstaining from the cocaine, OxyContin, and alcohol she had been using, her moods stabilized. It became apparent that she didn't have a mental health problem in addition to her addiction. When a person is getting off drugs or alcohol, it can take thirty to ninety days for the brain to clear and to get a true picture of their mental health.

One way to distinguish whether or not this is ADD or a drug-induced ADD look-a-like state is through clinical history. If someone had ADD symptoms before they ever used drugs, it is more likely a contributing factor. If they had no prior evidence of it, then it is more likely that their substance abuse caused their symptoms and waiting until they are clean for several months makes more sense in making the diagnosis.

Are you suffering from posttraumatic stress disorder? Your brain has more than one hundred billion brain cells, also called neurons. Throughout the day these neurons are either at rest or firing off electrical signals as a way to communicate with other neurons in order to spark your thoughts, behaviors, and emotions. They also fire off in high-stress situations. Let's say you are a soldier in Iraq and are always watching out for roadside bombs. The process of always having to be on guard causes your neurons to fire repeatedly and activates your brain's emotional centers. If you experience enough anxious or tense moments during your tour of duty, it can make your neurons fire faster, like a hairpin trigger.

When you return home, your neurons are still on guard, ready to fire with little provocation. Your son drops a plate and the crashing noise makes you flip out. The moving shadows in your bedroom make you bolt upright in the middle of the night. When your daughter bends down to pick up a shiny quarter on the street, you lunge and tackle her to keep her from touching it. This is because your brain is overly stimulated, and you may be more inclined to drink alcohol, take painkillers, or overeat as a way to soothe your brain.

This process of creating overactive neurons is called *kindling*. In lab experiments, researchers have tested this theory by passing an electrical current through nerve cells to get them to fire off. They have found that if they pass a current through the cell often enough and long enough, they can eventually lower the level of the electrical current and still get the cells to fire off. When this occurs, the nerve cells are said to be kindled. Having kindled neurons is one of the causes of overactivity in the brain. Learning to calm these kindled cells becomes an important part of unchaining your brain.

Are there signs of dementia? Dementia has been linked to an increased risk for addiction and compulsive behaviors. When elderly people who have lived their entire lives without a problem suddenly develop a problem, I often think that some form of dementia may be involved. Take my patient—let's call him Grandpa Joe—for example. He had been married to his high school sweetheart for forty years and had loving relationships with his grown daughter and her three children.

But when he turned seventy-three, Grandpa Joe's visits to his grandchildren took a very inappropriate turn. When his ten-year-old granddaughter sat on his lap, he found himself compelled to stroke her skin and felt himself getting sexually aroused. He eventually acted on his lustful yearnings and molested his granddaughter. His daughter found out and banished him from her house. That's when he decided to come to the Amen Clinics. Grandpa Joe's SPECT scans showed the classic signs of dementia, which include lowered overall brain function. Memory screening tests and a thorough evaluation confirmed the diagnosis.

Have you been exposed to environmental toxins? Common environmental toxins, such as mold, insecticides, tobacco smoke, paint, and phthalates (found in thousands of plastic products), pose a risk to brain function and increase the incidence of brain disorders that can look like ADD. Brain scans of indoor painters show some of the highest levels of brain damage. Any damage to the brain can increase your vulnerability to addiction.

In 2009, researchers from the National Institute of Environmental Health Sciences reported that women who use insecticides have a higher than normal risk of developing autoimmune diseases like rheumatoid arthritis or lupus. Autoimmune diseases are in essence brain diseases because it is your brain that tells your body's immune system to attack your own body. Some people with autoimmune diseases turn to substance abuse to cope with the chronic pain and other problems associated with their conditions.

2. Know your important health numbers.

Getting a thorough physical evaluation can help you uncover biological factors that might be contributing to your problem and that when corrected, may help you break free from your addiction. On the following page is a checklist of twenty important numbers we often test for in our patients.

20 IMPORTANT HEALTH NUMBERS
YOU NEED TO KNOW

1. Vitamin D level
2. Omega-3 fatty acids level
3. Hormone levels
      o   thyroid (TSH and free T3)
      o   testosterone (for men and women)
      o   estrogen and progesterone (for women)
      o   DHEA-S level
4. HgA1c
5. Fasting blood sugar
6. Insulin level
7. Complete blood count (CBC)
8. Comprehensive metabolic panel
9. Two-hour glucose tolerance test (if hypoglycemia symptoms are present)
10. Cholesterol
11. C-reactive protein
12. Homocysteine
13. Blood pressure
14. The twelve most common modifiable risks you may have
15. Number of hours you sleep
16. BMI
17. Daily caloric needs
18. Daily caloric intake
19. Heavy metal toxicity
20. How many hidden food allergies you have

Vitamin D level. Vitamin deficiencies can harm your brain and increase your vulnerability for out-of-control behavior. Get a blood test called 25-hydroxy vitamin D to check your vitamin D level, and if it is low, get more sunshine and/or take a vitamin D3 supplement to get it in the optimal range.

Low: less than 30
Optimal: 50–90
High: over 90

Omega-3 fatty acids level. Omega-3 fatty acids are critical for optimal brain function. They are healthy fats that come from foods like wild salmon, avocados, and walnuts. Scientific evidence suggests that low levels of omega-3 fatty acids play a role in substance abuse. The test we use at the Amen Clinics involves a simple finger prick to get a few drops of blood. If levels are low, eat more foods rich in omega-3 and/or take a daily fish oil supplement. We have found that almost all of our patients are low unless they focus on eating fish or take an omega-3 supplement.

Hormone levels (thyroid, DHEA-S, testosterone, estrogen, and progesterone). Most people think "hormones" are only involved in reproductive issues. Not true. Hormones are essential for health and vitality in both men and women, and it is the brain that controls all the hormones in your body. Your hormones all work together to achieve beautiful balance, but if a single hormone isn't working hard enough or is working too hard, it can throw your whole system off balance. Imbalanced hormones clearly impact how the brain works and can contribute to impulse problems and compulsive behaviors.

Having problems with your thyroid can cause symptoms that make you want to self-medicate with food, drugs, alcohol, or thrilling behaviors. An overactive thyroid can mimic symptoms of anxiety that make you want to drink alcohol or take painkillers to calm down. Low thyroid levels cause your body's systems to function at a slower speed, which may drive you seek out stimulating substances or behaviors. Having low thyroid levels also decreases overall brain activity, which can impair your thinking, judgment, and self-control.

Dr. Marvin "Rick" Sponaugle, founder and medical director of the Sponaugle Wellness Institute & Addiction Treatment Center, which has successfully treated over five thousand addicted patients, insists that the role of hormones in addiction can't be overlooked. "We have successfully proven that over 90 percent of addicted patients self-medicate with drugs and alcohol in their attempt to balance their brain chemistry and feel more normal," he writes in a paper entitled *Anti-aging/Longevity Medicine Reduces the Prevalence of Alcoholism and Drug Addiction*. "Patients utilize drugs and alcohol either to stimulate under-active brain regions or relax over-active brain systems. The aberrant electrical activity in the addicted patient's brain is typically caused by inherited or acquired biochemical and hormonal deficiencies."

For women, Sponaugle points to declining levels of progesterone, a calming hormone, during perimenopause as a source for anxiety and insomnia that drives women to abuse drugs and alcohol. Women who normally drink a glass of wine with dinner will progress to a couple of bottles of wine at night, he writes. He claims this is the case with more than 40 percent of the middle-aged females at his treatment facility. Other women in perimenopause will turn to drugs like Vicodin or OxyContin to calm their brains. Sponaugle has found that when female patients use hormone replacement therapy, their cravings for these substances subside.

Having low testosterone levels for men or women has been associated with low energy and depression, both of which may drive a person to self-medicate. Low levels of the hormone DHEA-S can produce some of the same problems.

Testing hormone levels involves a blood test. Have your doctor check your free T3 and TSH levels to check for hypo-thyroidism or hyperthyroidism and treat as necessary to normalize.

Also have your physician test your DHEA-S, testosterone, and (for women only) estrogen and progesterone levels. If your hormone levels are off, consider balancing them with hormone replacement therapy.

HgAlc. This test shows your average blood sugar levels over the past two to three months and is used to diagnose diabetes and prediabetes. Having diabetes has been shown to lower impulse control. Here is a look at what the A1c numbers indicate:

Normal: 4.0–5.6
Prediabetes: 5.7–6.4
Diabetes: 6.5 or higher

Fasting blood sugar. This test usually requires that you fast for about eight hours prior to having your blood drawn. It evaluates your blood sugar levels solely for the day when you have your blood drawn. Here is what the levels mean:

Normal: 70–99 mg/dL
Prediabetes: 100–125 mg/dL
Diabetes: 126 mg/dL or higher

Insulin level. This test is used to diagnose insulin resistance, a condition that raises your risk for diabetes.

Complete blood count (CBC). The CBC is used to screen for a wide variety of disorders, including anemia and infection, which negatively impact brain function.

Comprehensive metabolic panel. Have your doctor order this blood test to evaluate the status of your kidneys, liver, electrolytes, and more.

Two-hour glucose tolerance test. This is used to test for diabetes and reactive hypoglycemia. It involves drinking a glucose solution, then having blood drawn at several intervals during a two-hour period.

Cholesterol. Having high levels of cholesterol is associated with an increased risk for heart disease and dementia later in life. Both of these conditions decrease brain function. Make sure your doctor checks your total cholesterol level as well as your HDL (good cholesterol), LDL (bad cholesterol), and triglycerides (a form of fat). Optimal levels are as follows:

Total cholesterol: less than 200
HDL: 60 or higher
LDL: less than 100
Triglycerides: less than 150

C-reactive protein. This is a measure of inflammation that your doctor can check with a simple blood test. Elevated inflammation is associated with diseases and conditions that affect brain health.

Homocysteine level. This is another marker of inflammation.

Blood pressure. High blood pressure increases your risk for heart disease and stroke. Have your doctor check your blood pressure to determine if it is high. Here is how to interpret the numbers:

Optimal: below 120 over 80
Prehypertension: 120–139 over 80–89
Hypertension: 140 (or above) over 90 (or above)

The twelve most common modifiable health risks. Know how many of the twelve most common preventable causes of death you have...then decrease them.

1. Smoking
2. High blood pressure
3. BMI indicating overweight or obese
4. Physical inactivity
5. High fasting blood glucose
6. High LDL cholesterol
7. Alcohol abuse (accidents, violence, cirrhosis, liver disease, cancer, stroke, heart disease, hypertension)
8. Low omega-3 fatty acids
9. High dietary saturated fat intake
10. Low polyunsaturated fat intake
11. High dietary salt intake
12. Low intake of fruits and vegetables

Number of hours you sleep. Don't fool yourself into thinking you need only a few hours of sleep. Sleep deprivation reduces brain function and lowers impulse control. You can read more about this in Chapter 9: Boost Your Brain to Get Control. Here are the average sleep requirements by age:

Age Range	Number of Hours of Sleep
1–3 years old	12–14 hours
3–5 years old	11–13 hours
5–12 years old	10–11 hours
13–19 years old	9 hours
Adults	7–8 hours
Seniors	7–8 hours

Body mass index (BMI). Your BMI indicates whether or not you have a healthy weight. This is important because being overweight or obese is associated with having a smaller brain and increases your risk for many medical conditions. To calculate your BMI, use the BMI Calculator at www.amenclincis.com/cybcyb or use the following equation:

$$\textit{Weight in pounds} \times \textit{703/height in inches}^2$$

Here's how to interpret your BMI:

Underweight: below 18.5
Normal: 18.5–25
Overweight: 25–29
Obese: 30–39
Morbidly obese: 40 and over

Daily caloric needs to maintain current body weight. To find out your basic calorie needs without exercise, which is referred to as your resting basal metabolic rate (BMR), use the following equation:

Women: *655 + (4.35 × weight in pounds) + (4.7 × height in inches) − (4.7 × age in years)*

Men: *66 + (6.23 × weight in pounds) + (12.7 × height in inches) −*
(6.8 × age in years)

Take that number and multiply it by the appropriate number below.

1.2 – if you are sedentary (little or no exercise)

1.375 – if you are lightly active (light exercise/sports 1–3 days a week)

1.55 – if you are moderately active (moderate exercise/ sports 3–5 days a week)

1.75 – if you are very active (hard exercise/sports 6–7 days a week)

1.9 – if you are extra active (very hard exercise/sports and a physical job or strength training twice a day)

Daily caloric intake (don't lie to yourself). Keep track of everything you eat and drink along with their calorie counts to find out how much you are truly eating each day. It would be very helpful for you to keep a daily journal for at least a week.

Heavy metal toxicity. A few hair samples is all that is required for this test, which can show if you have high levels of dangerous heavy metals in your system.

How many hidden food allergies you have. Having allergies or sensitivities to certain foods or food additives can alter the way your brain functions and lead to physical, emotional, behavioral, and learning problems. Headaches or migraines, joint pain, chronic sinus problems, gastrointestinal issues, sleep problems, lack of concentration, anxiety, aggression, and violence are just some of the symptoms associated with food sensitivities and allergies. A person might turn to addictive substances as a way to deal with these issues.

Peanuts, milk, eggs, soy, fish, shellfish, tree nuts, and wheat account for 90 percent of all food-allergic reactions. Other foods commonly associated with allergies include corn, chocolate, tea, coffee, sugar, yeast, citrus fruits, pork, rye, beef, tomato, and barley. Food additives like MSG and red dye can also cause problems for some people. Surprisingly, the foods we are allergic to are often the ones we crave the most.

When food allergies are suspected, I order a Delayed Immunoglobin G (IgG) Food Allergy Test, which tests for ninety-three foods. It involves a simple blood draw. Another way to evaluate food allergies is to do an elimination diet. I often will ask people to read the work of Doris Rapp, MD, who has written about food allergies and mental illness for decades.

Other tests based on your history and individual profile. Depending on your particular needs, other tests may be warranted.

3. Family History

Your family history influences your risk, which is why a good evaluation must include a detailed family history. If your family tree is filled with people who are overeaters, alcoholics, drug abusers, or gamblers, chances are you have a heightened risk for following in their footsteps. If one or both of your parents has a problem, you are certainly more likely to have a problem yourself.

Psychological Evaluation

It is also critical to evaluate all relevant psychological issues, such as negative thinking patterns, past emotional trauma, and readiness to change.

Negative thinking. After treating thousands of patients with addictions, we have realized that negative thinking patterns can crush your efforts to change your habits. I call these thoughts ANTs (automatic negative thoughts). ANTs are the thoughts that enter your head, make you feel bad, prevent you from adopting healthy brain habits, and keep you chained to your addiction. Correcting these negative thought patterns is an essential step in the healing process. In Chapter 12: Kill the Addiction ANTs That Infest Your Brain and Keep You in Chains, you will learn how to talk back to the lies you tell yourself so you can change your thinking and unchain your brain.

Past emotional trauma. Amanda, sixteen, was sexually abused by her uncle when she was eleven years old. But she never talked about it and did the best she could to bury the hurt deep inside her. This terrible event drove Amanda to drink alcohol to deal with her unresolved emotional issues. When Amanda entered a rehab facility, she finally opened up about the sexual assault and was able to get the counseling she needed to process her feelings.

Amanda's story is very common among people with addictions. In fact, a 2002 study in the *Journal of Substance Abuse Treatment* found that a stunning 81 percent of the women and 69 percent of the men in a treatment facility reported past physical and sexual abuse. The abuse started at a median age of thirteen for the women and eleven for the men. In order to unchain your brain, you must deal with any past emotional issues.

Readiness to change. One of the most important parts of any evaluation is determining how ready you are to change. Have you accepted that you have a problem, or are you still in denial? Do you understand what you need to do in order to change, or do you need help learning what to do? Are you able to work on your recovery from home, or do you need more structured care? Are you highly motivated to change, or do you need other people to keep you motivated to stay on the right track? Knowing how ready you are can help you find the best treatment options for you.

Social Evaluation

When we evaluate patients with addiction, we always take their social situation and recovery environment into consideration. Do you have a good social support system, or do the people around you create a lot of stress in your life? Are the people in your life likely to trigger your desire to slip back into your old habits? For example, if you are trying to break free from your addiction to cigarettes, does your spouse smoke, which will make it very hard for you to abstain? Are your friends smokers? Do you work in a bar or nightclub where patrons smoke?

It is also important to understand the stresses in your life. Are your relationships troubled? Is money a problem? Is your job too demanding? Are you caring for an elderly parent or sick child?

I also ask my patients about their daily habits and participation in thrilling behaviors that might be altering their brain chemistry. Are you constantly texting or checking your Facebook page? Do you play a lot of video games, watch a lot of TV, or spend a lot of time on your computer? Taking stock of your social situation can help you navigate your recovery.

Spiritual Evaluation

In previous chapters, I talked about how important it is to figure out what your life means to you and why you want to change. Unearthing what is driving you to change is an essential part of a good evaluation. It can take some time and self-reflection to discover your true sense of spirituality but it should be addressed.

UNCHAIN YOUR BRAIN CHECKLIST

- ✓ Getting a comprehensive evaluation that looks at all four pillar—biological, psychological, social, and spiritual—is critical to healing.

- ✓ Seek out an addiction professional, treatment program, or support group that examines all four pillars and how they are involved in your problem.

- ✓ Evaluate your brain health.

- ✓ Know your important health numbers.

- ✓ Examine your family history.

- ✓ Evaluate your thinking patterns.

- ✓ Face up to past emotional trauma.

- ✓ Gauge your readiness to change.

- ✓ Take stock of your social situation and recovery environment.

- ✓ Discover what your life means to you and why you want to change.

Chapter 8

Step #3

KNOW YOUR BRAIN TYPE

Learn the Six Different Types of Addiction
When it comes to treatment for addiction, one size does NOT fit all.

Leigh, forty-two, couldn't stop thinking about gambling. The minute he woke up, he powered up his computer to check the spreads on that day's sporting events. At work, he was easily distracted and had trouble concentrating because he was constantly checking the scores and planning his next bets. On a single game, he would often bet not only on which team would win based on the point spread, but also on halftime scores, individual player stats, and more. He came to our clinics because his wife was threatening to divorce him if he didn't stop gambling and because he worried incessantly and held grudges.

Randall, fifty-one, started smoking when he was sixteen. He thought it made him look cool, and it helped him focus on his classwork. Considering he was in jeopardy of failing several classes because he had trouble finishing assignments on time, he felt like he needed all the help he could get. His troubles followed him into adulthood, and he got fired from several jobs for being disorganized and chronically late for work. When his mother got lung cancer after a lifetime of smoking, he decided to quit. He woke up every morning with good intentions, but if he saw someone else light up, he couldn't resist reaching for a cigarette. Randall brought his son to us for school-related issues, similar to the problems he had experienced growing up. When he saw how much his son improved on treatment, he decided to get an evaluation as well.

Shanice, thirty-three, always had a sweet tooth. As a child, she would sprinkle sugar on her Lucky Charms, put gummy bears and chocolate chips on top of her ice cream, and dip her toast in maple syrup. As an adult, her taste buds didn't change. She still craved sweets and would nibble on cookies on the way to work, munch on candy bars after lunch, and eat at least three scoops of ice cream late at night. Shanice was plagued by negative thoughts and whenever she felt stressed, she would turn to treats for comfort. The extra calories had added forty pounds to her body, and she hated the way she looked. In her twenties, she developed bulimia in an effort to keep the weight off in spite of her overindulgences. Shanice came to see us to deal with her emotions following the death of her father, who had been an alcoholic for most of his life.

Danielle, nineteen, was a college student who grew up in a family of depressed people. Both of her parents struggled with mood problems, and Danielle began having feelings of despair as early as junior high. By the time she got to college, she was tired of feeling blue and having little energy. While home for the holidays, Danielle found some OxyContin left over from her dad's root canal surgery and decided to try one. The drug made her feel happy and truly alive for the first time in her life. After the effects wore off, she couldn't wait to feel that way again. She took the rest of the pills back to college and when they were gone, she started buying OxyContin from a guy at college. When her regular supplier wasn't around, she bought it from a new guy at school who turned out to be an undercover cop. Danielle got arrested and wound up in court-ordered drug treatment with David, who ordered a SPECT study from us.

Kim, twenty-five, felt nervous all the time and was always under a lot of stress from her job in advertising. She had a lot of unexplained headaches, stomachaches, and muscle tension. She had smoked marijuana in college to help her calm down, but her new employer did employee drug testing, and she didn't want to get fired so she started drinking instead. Typically, she couldn't wait until quitting time so she could stop at the bar down the street for a few drinks to unwind. Even though she drank every day, she never felt drunk so she didn't think she had an addiction. When she came to our clinics at the urging of her boyfriend, who was irritated by her anxiety, we found that her brain showed clear damage from alcohol.

Scott, thirty-two, couldn't get enough of his video games. From the minute he got home from work, he would hit the gaming console and often forgot to eat because he was so engrossed in his game. On many weekends, he played so much he wouldn't leave his apartment. Other activities bored him, even things he used to enjoy like playing basketball or going to the movies with his girlfriend. If his girlfriend complained about his constant gaming, Scott would scream at her to leave him alone. His girlfriend noticed that ever since he was involved in a car accident, he had developed a hot temper, had trouble remembering their friends' names, and had difficulty learning to use the remote control for their new TV. When his outbursts escalated, she threatened to leave him if he didn't get help. That's when he showed up in our office.

Not All Addicts are the Same

Leigh, Randall, Shanice, Danielle, Kim, and Scott all struggled with addictions. Yet, they all had very different clinical presentations and brain patterns.

Leigh was a compulsive addict. He couldn't stop thinking about gambling. His brain SPECT study showed too much activity in the anterior cingulate gyrus (ACG), likely due to low levels of the neurotransmitter serotonin. Taking the natural supplements 5-HTP, inositol, and saffron, which is in my Serotonin Mood Support supplement, boosted serotonin levels and helped him overcome his constant worrying. Combined with psychotherapy and attendance at a gambling support group, he was finally able to curb his gambling.

Randall was an impulsive addict. He couldn't control his urge to smoke. His SPECT scans showed classic signs of attention deficit disorder (ADD), including low activity in the prefrontal cortex, likely due to low levels of dopamine. Low PFC activity explained why he had trouble supervising his own behavior. On medication to treat ADD plus hypnosis, he was better able to control his impulses and stop smoking.

Shanice was an impulsive-compulsive addict. She had features of both impulsivity and compulsivity. Her SPECT scans showed both an overactive ACG and an underactive PFC, likely due to low levels of both serotonin and dopamine. In my research, I have discovered that this pattern is common in children and grandchildren of alcoholics. On treatment to raise both serotonin and dopamine, Shanice finally got control of her cravings for sweets. Combined with psychotherapy, she was able to overcome her bulimia and finally lose weight and keep it off.

Danielle was a sad or emotional addict. She medicated her feelings of sadness with drugs. Her SPECT scans showed increased activity in the deep limbic system. With a combination of the natural supplement SAMe (found in my SAMe Mood & Movement Support supplement), exercise, dietary changes, and therapy, Danielle managed to kick her OxyContin habit for good.

Kim was an anxious addict. She medicated her underlying anxiety with alcohol. Her SPECT scans showed too much activity in the basal ganglia. With a treatment plan that included relaxation techniques combined with the natural supplements B6, magnesium, and GABA (found in my GABA Calming Support supplement), she felt more calm and no longer felt the need to turn to alcohol.

Scott was a temporal lobe addict. His hot temper and poor memory were causing both relational and learning issues. He lost himself in the video games as a way to soothe himself. His SPECT scans showed evidence of a head injury to his temporal lobes, likely from the car accident, in addition to low activity in the PFC. On anticonvulsant medication to normalize his temporal lobes, combined with ADD medication to boost his prefrontal cortex and increased exercise, his violent outbursts diminished and his obsession with video gaming waned.

Compulsive Addict
Hyperfrontal

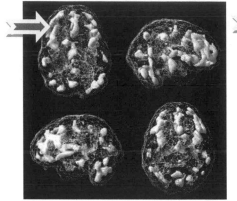

Increased anterior cingulate activity

Impulsive Addict
Hypofrontal

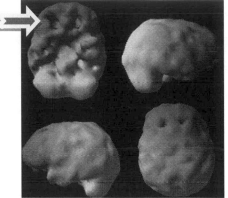

Low prefrontal cortex activity

Impulsive-Compulsive Addict—Both Hyperfrontal and Hypofrontal

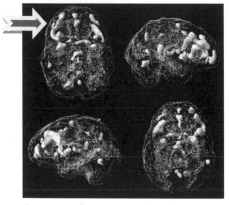

Increased anterior cingulate activity

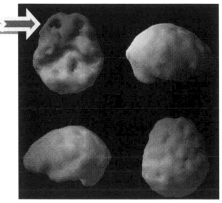

Low prefrontal cortex activity

Sad Addict

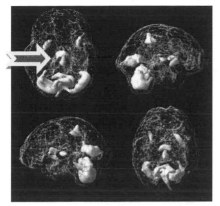

Increased deep limbic activity

Anxious Addict

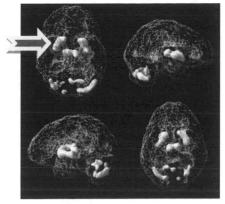

Increased basal ganglia activity

Temporal Lobe Addict

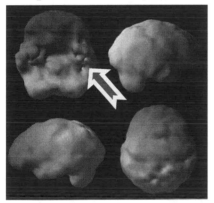

Low temporal lobe activity and overall decreased activity consistent with toxicity from drugs or alcohol

Summary of the Amen Clinics Six Types of Addicts

Based on our brain imaging work with tens of thousands of patients, I have identified six types of addicts based on brain patterns. Knowing which type you are is essential to finding the best treatment plan for your own specific needs. To help you find your type, take the Unchain Your Brain Master Questionnaire in Appendix A or take the extended version online at www.amenclinics.com.

Type 1: Compulsive Addicts

People with this type have trouble shifting their attention and tend to get stuck on thoughts of gambling, Internet porn, food, or some other substance or behavior. Regardless of what these people are addicted to, the thinking pattern and basic mechanism are the same. They tend to get stuck or locked into one course of action and have trouble seeing options.

The most common brain SPECT finding in this type is increased anterior cingulate gyrus activity, which is most commonly caused by low brain serotonin levels. High-protein diets and stimulants, such as Ritalin, usually make this type worse. Interventions to boost serotonin in the brain are generally the most helpful. From a supplement standpoint, 5-HTP, inositol, and saffron (found in my Serotonin Mood Support supplement), L-tryptophan, or St. John's wort are helpful, as are the serotonin-enhancing medications, such as Prozac, Zoloft, and Lexapro.

Behavioral interventions that boost serotonin to help compulsive addicts:

- Exercise to allow more of the serotonin precursor L-tryptophan to get into the brain.
- If you get an addiction-oriented thought in your head more than three times, do something to distract yourself.
- Make a list of ten things you can do instead of the addictive behavior so you can distract yourself.
- People with this type always do better with choices, rather than edicts. Do not tell them what they are going to do; give them choices.
- Avoid automatically opposing others or saying "no," even to yourself.
- If you have trouble sleeping, try a glass of warm milk with a teaspoon of vanilla and a few drops of the natural sweetener stevia.

Type 2: Impulsive Addicts

People with this type have trouble with impulse control even though they may start each day with the intention of refraining from their addictive behaviors. The most common SPECT finding for this type is low activity in the PFC, likely due to low levels of dopamine. The PFC acts as the brain's supervisor and is involved in judgment, impulse control, planning, and follow through. When it is underactive, people can be easily distracted, bored, inattentive, and impulsive. This type is often seen in conjunction with ADD and is more common in males.

High-carbohydrate diets and serotonin-enhancing medications, such as Prozac, Zoloft, or Lexapro, or supplements, such as 5-HTP, usually make this type worse. Interventions to boost dopamine in the brain are generally the most helpful. From a supplement standpoint, green tea and rhodiola (found in my Focus & Energy Optimizer supplement), and l-tyrosine are helpful, as are stimulant medications, such as Adderall and Ritalin, which are commonly used to treat ADD.

Behavioral interventions that boost dopamine to help impulsive addicts:

- Exercise, which helps increase blood flow and dopamine in the brain—especially doing an exercise you love.
- Clear focus—write your goals in your One Page Miracle and display it where you can see it every day.
- Outside supervision—have someone you trust check in with you on a regular basis to help you stay focused on your goals.
- Avoid impulsively saying "yes" to offers of alcohol, drugs, food, or whatever your particular addiction is. Practice saying, "No."

147

Type 3: Impulsive-Compulsive Addicts

People with this type have a combination of both impulsive and compulsive features. This type is common in people with bulimia. The brain SPECT scans tend to show low activity in the PFC (associated with impulsivity, likely due to low dopamine levels) and too much activity in the anterior cingulate gyrus (associated with compulsivity and low serotonin levels). This pattern is common in the children and grandchildren of alcoholics.

Using treatments that boost either serotonin or dopamine alone usually makes the problem worse. For example, using supplements or medications that increase serotonin only calms the compulsions but makes the impulsivity worse. Taking supplements or medications that raise dopamine levels only improves impulse control but increases the compulsive behaviors. In my experience, I have found that people with this type do best with treatments that raise both serotonin and dopamine. For example, combining green tea (for dopamine) and 5-HTP (for serotonin) or Ritalin (for dopamine) and Prozac (for serotonin) can be helpful.

Behavioral interventions that boost both serotonin and dopamine to help impulsive-compulsive addicts:

- Exercise.
- Set goals.
- Avoid automatically opposing others or saying "no," even to yourself.
- Avoid impulsively saying "yes."
- Have options.
- Distract yourself if you get a thought stuck in your head.

Type 4: Sad or Emotional Addicts

People with this type often use alcohol, marijuana, painkillers, or food to medicate underlying feelings of depression, boredom, or loneliness. This type is more commonly seen in women. For some people, these feelings come and go with the seasons and tend to worsen in winter. Others experience mild feelings of chronic sadness, called dysthymia. Still others suffer from more serious depressions. The typical SPECT findings associated with this type are hyperactivity in the deep limbic system and low activity in the PFC.

When depression is mild, it can often be treated with natural supplements like SAMe (found in my SAMe Mood & Movement Support supplement), in addition to exercise, dietary changes, and psychotherapy. For more serious cases, antidepressant medication may be required. Taking vitamin D can also be beneficial for people with depression, especially for people whose addictions worsen or are triggered during the winter months, a condition called seasonal affective disorder (SAD).

Having low levels of vitamin D, known as the "sunshine" vitamin, has been associated with depression, memory problems, obesity, heart disease, and immune suppression. Vitamin D deficiencies are becoming more common in our society for two reasons: we are wearing more sunscreen and spending more time indoors. In an Amen Clinics weight-loss study completed in 2010, we tested the vitamin D levels or more than thirty participants. I was shocked to discover that everybody's levels were low, and this study took place in sunny southern California!

Other natural treatments for depression include bright light therapy, which has also been found to effectively treat SAD, the natural supplement SAMe (in dosages of 400 to 1,600 mg), and the hormone DHEA. Be careful with SAMe if you have ever experienced a manic episode, and take it early in the day as it has energizing properties and may interfere with sleep. DHEA is a master hormone that has been found to be low in people with depression and obesity.

Behavioral interventions that boost mood to help sad, or emotional, addicts:

- Exercise to increase blood flow and multiple neuro-transmitters in the brain.

- Kill the ANTs (automatic negative thoughts) that steal your happiness.
- Write down five things you are grateful for every day (this has been shown to increase your level of happiness in just three weeks).
- Volunteer to help others, which helps to get you outside of yourself and less focused on your own internal problems.
- Surround yourself with great smells, such as lavender.
- Try melatonin to help you sleep.
- Work to improve your relationships.

Type 5: Anxious Addicts

People with this type tend to use alcohol, marijuana, painkillers, sleeping pills, or food to medicate underlying feelings of anxiety, tension, nervousness, and fear. More commonly seen in women, this type tends to suffer physical symptoms of anxiety, such as muscle tension, headaches, stomachaches, nail biting, heart palpitations, and shortness of breath. People with this type tend to predict the worst and may be excessively shy or easily startled. The SPECT finding that correlates to this type is too much activity in the basal ganglia, likely due to low levels of GABA.

Interventions that boost GABA are generally the most helpful, and include taking B6, magnesium, and GABA (found in my GABA Calming Support supplement). Relaxation therapies can also be helpful to calm this area of the brain.

Behavioral interventions that boost GABA and calm the brain to help anxious addicts:

- Exercise.
- Try relaxation exercises, such as:
  o meditation
  o prayer
  o hypnosis
  o deep diaphragmatic breathing exercises
  o hand-warming techniques

- Kill the anxious ANTs.
- For sleep, try hypnosis or my Restful Sleep formula that contains melatonin, GABA, valerian, magnesium, and B6.

Type 6: Temporal Lobe Addicts

People with this type tend to have problems with temper, mood swings, learning problems, and memory problems. Abnormal activity in the temporal lobes is commonly due to past head injuries, infections, a lack of oxygen, or exposure to environmental toxins, or it may be inherited. The SPECT findings are decreased activity in the temporal lobes. Sometimes we also see excessive increased activity.

Treatments to stabilize activity in the temporal lobes may involve boosting the calming neurotransmitter GABA or the memory and learning neurotransmitter acetylcholine, a higher-protein diet, and completely eliminating sugar. Ways to boost GABA include using supplements, such as our GABA Calming Support, which contains GABA and magnesium, or anticonvulsant or anti-seizure medications, like Lamictal. Ways to boost acetylcholine in the brain, which can help with memory and learning, include using either supplements, such as huperzine A and acetyl-l-carnitine (contained in our Brain & Memory Power Boost formula), or medications, such as Aricept or Exelon. Together, these strategies can help with temper control, mood stability, learning, and memory.

Behavioral interventions that normalize temporal lobe activity and boost dopamine to help temporal lobe addicts:

- New learning.
- Preventing further head injuries.

Do You Have More Than One Type?

Having more than one type is common, and it just means that you may need a combination of interventions to help you unchain your brain. Type 3 Impulsive-Compulsive Addicts is actually a combination of Type 1 Compulsive Addicts and Type 2 Impulsive Addicts. It is common to have Type 1 mixed with Type 4 Sad or Emotional Addicts or with Type 5 Anxious Addicts. In those cases, we may mix 5-HTP for Type 1 with SAMe for Type 4 or GABA for Type 5. Again, it is always smart to discuss these options with your healthcare provider or treatment program. If he or she does not know much about natural treatments, consult a naturopath or a physician trained in integrative medicine or natural treatments.

SUMMARY CHART OF THE AMEN CLINICS SIX TYPES OF ADDICTS

Type	Symptoms	Brain Findings/ Neurotransmitter Issue	*Supplements* & **Medications**
1. Compulsive Addicts	overfocused, worrying, trouble letting go of hurts	increased AC (anterior cingulate)/low serotonin	*Serotonin Mood Support (5-HTP, inositol, saffron), or St. John's wort* SSRIs, such as Prozac, Zoloft, or Lexapro
2. Impulsive Addicts	impulsivity, bored, easily distracted	low PFC (prefrontal cortex)/low dopamine	*Focus & Energy Optimizer (green tea, rhodiola) or L-tyrosine* Stimulants such as Adderall or Ritalin
3. Impulsive-Compulsive Addicts	combination of types 1 and 2	high AC plus low PFC/low serotonin and dopamine	*5-HTP plus green tea and rhodiola* SSRI plus phentermine or stimulant
4. Sad or Emotional Addicts	sad or depressed mood, winter blues, carbohydrate cravings, loss of interest, sleeps a lot, low energy, self-medicates to improve mood	high limbic activity, low PFC/check vitamin D and DHEA levels	*SAMe Mood & Movement Support, vitamin D, or DHEA if needed* Wellbutrin

Type	Symptoms	Brain Findings/ Neurotransmitter Issue	*Supplements* & **Medications**
5. Anxious Addicts	anxious, tense, nervous, predicts the worst, self-medicates to calm	high basal ganglia/low GABA levels	*GABA Calming Support (GABA, B6, magnesium)* Anticonvulsants, such as Topamax, Neurontin
6. Temporal Lobe Addicts	temper problems, mood instability, memory problems, learning disabilities	abnormal TL	*GABA Calming Support (GABA, B6, magnesium) for calming, or Brain & Memory Power Boost (huperzine A, acetyl-l-carnitine, vinpocetine, ginkgo) for memory* Anticonvulsants, such as Lamictal for mood stability, Aricept or Namenda for memory enhancement

Male vs. Female Brains: Gender-Specific Addictions and Treatments

One of the most fascinating things I have learned from looking at more than 57,000 brain scans is that male and female brains are NOT the same. Actually, when it comes to the brain it is hard to find areas that are NOT affected by gender. For example, the prefrontal cortex is larger in women. This is the most human, thoughtful part of the brain and when it is low people are more likely to have trouble with impulse control and excitement-seeking behavior, hence why guys tend to do more stupid things, like jump out of perfectly good airplanes, much more than women. Men have a larger amygdala, an area in your temporal lobes that has been implicated in aggression. Women have a larger hippocampus, a major memory structure in the brain, which is why she is likely to remember every bad thing you ever did.

Some of the differences between the male and female brain can affect what you get addicted to and why. For example, women are about twice as likely as men to suffer from anxiety and depression. They are also at higher risk for sexual assault, domestic violence, and childhood physical abuse, which can contribute to stress, anxiety, and depression. Because of this, women are more likely to self-medicate their feelings of sadness or nervousness with alcohol, prescription painkillers, marijuana, or a combination of drugs and alcohol.

Males, on the other hand, are more likely to be diagnosed with ADD, which makes them more impulsive. They tend to seek out stimulating substances, such as cocaine, methamphetamine, or high doses of caffeine, and thrilling behaviors, such as video gaming, viewing Internet pornography, or voyeurism. In many cases, taking some form of stimulants makes them feel so amped up that they then feel the need to drink alcohol or smoke pot as a way to relax.

Tweens, Teens, and Seniors: Getting the Right Help for Your Age

When kids get sick, we take them to the pediatrician. When women go through menopause, they see a gynecologist. When grandparents experience memory problems, they make an appointment with a specialist in Alzheimer's and age-related conditions. With addicts however, we send them all to cookie-cutter treatment programs that are geared to adults, and typically to adult males. And while these treatment programs can be very effective for some people, they don't necessarily address the special needs of some individuals.

Based on our brain imaging work, we have found that the brains of young people are very different from adult brains and much more vulnerable to addiction. Until the age of twenty-five, young brains are going through a process called myelinization that wraps neurons in a protective coating that renders them ten to one hundred times more efficient. The prefrontal cortex is the last part of the brain to undergo this process, leaving tweens and teens with a tendency for impulse control problems. This is why adolescents are much more likely to say, "Okay" when a friend offers them beer, pot, methamphetamine, cocaine, Ecstasy, or Ritalin. I often tell parents to be patient and work to keep their keep their kids safe until they are twenty-five.

I recently had a discussion with a long-time friend of mine whose son I saw when he was a teen. He was a mess with school and drug problems. I put him in a drug treatment program and put him on our brain healthy strategies. It helped, but the mother was still very concerned. I preached about patience and safety to his mother. Her son is now twenty-eight, engaged, employed, and back in school, but this time with his own motivation.

In my practice, I have also found that young people who have problems with addiction often have co-occurring disorders, such as depression, anxiety, bipolar disorder, or ADD. The problem is that in traditional treatment programs, these problems can be hard to diagnose. In many cases, the effects of substance abuse can mimic the symptoms associated with mental health conditions. Similarly, hormonal changes in teens can cause moodiness, sadness, and distractibility. This is why brain imaging is so helpful in working with young addicts. Brain scans can help determine whether problem behaviors are just a normal part of growing up, a symptom of addiction, or the result of underlying brain dysfunction.

When youngsters under the age of fifteen get addicted to drugs, alcohol, gambling, or food, they are damaging circuits that aren't fully formed. Anything that disrupts the myelinization process can potentially permanently change the brain in a negative way. This can permanently rewire the brain, increasing the risk for relapse throughout life. When you hurt the PFC, it negatively affects the cerebellum (at the back bottom part of the brain, which is involved in processing speed, or how quickly you can think). For young people who want to break free from addiction, it is critical to strengthen the PFC. Intense exercise, focused goals, and external supervision are key to the healing process.

How can a career woman who has been a social drinker all her life progress into alcoholism after going through menopause? How can a kind grandfather who has been happily married to the same woman for forty-five years suddenly develop a penchant for Internet porn? How can a successful entrepreneur who spent his entire life building his business gamble away all his savings after selling the business and retiring?

Elderly people are not immune to addiction. In fact, certain age-related conditions can set the stage for the onset of addiction in the graying population. For example, developing frontal lobe dementia can derail the PFC and lead to impulse control problems. Heart disease is the number-one killer in America, and having coronary artery bypass grafting surgery (CABG) has been associated with subsequent cognitive impairment. In addition, many common prescription medications can alter brain chemistry and make older individuals who used to have healthy self-control fall victim to addiction.

Anything that takes the PFC offline allows the limbic brain to take over. When the drive circuits take control of your brain, it raises your risk for addiction. In elderly people with addictions, it is very important to treat any underlying memory loss and to review all medications being taken. Following heart bypass surgery, it is critical to adopt a brain healthy program to counteract the effects of cognitive decline. Changing hormones in mid-life can negatively affect the brains of both men and women, leaving them more vulnerable to problems.

UNCHAIN YOUR BRAIN CHECKLIST

✓ Remember that all addicts are NOT the same—the Amen Clinics has identified six types of addicts.

✓ The six types of addicts are:
   1. Type 1 Compulsive Addicts
   2. Type 2 Impulsive Addicts
   3. Type 3 Impulsive-Compulsive Addicts
   4. Type 4 Anxious Addicts
   5. Type 5 Sad or Emotional Addicts
   6. Type 6 Temporal Lobe Addicts.

✓ Take the Unchain Your Brain Master Questionnaire in Appendix A to find out which type of addict you may be.

✓ Remember that when it comes to treatment, one size does NOT fit all.

✓ Understanding the role gender plays in addiction can help you unchain your brain.

✓ If you are a young person with addiction, you must work to strengthen and protect your PFC.

✓ If you are older, you must treat underlying brain and memory problems and be careful with medications.

Chapter 9

Step #4

BOOST YOUR BRAIN
TO GET CONTROL

And Prevent Lasting Memory
Problems and Brain Damage

*You are not stuck with the brain you have. You can make it better,
and we can prove it.*

W hy should you care about boosting your brain? Because it is
your brain that controls everything you do. It is the
supercomputer that helps you get and keep friends and romantic
partners, get into college, land a great job, start and grow your own
business, learn to play the drums, write a hit song, make the
basketball team, and be a good dad, mom, husband, wife,
girlfriend, boyfriend, son, daughter, in-law, or grandparent.

- It is your brain that gives you the social skills to land a date
  with that special someone or that makes you blurt out
  something inappropriate that makes them say "No, thanks"
  when you ask them out.

- It is your brain that makes you loving and reliable so your
  family life is stress-free or that makes you irritable and
  unpredictable, which creates tension at home.

- It is your brain that allows you to do a great job and meet
  your deadlines at work so you get a promotion and a better
  salary, or that makes you turn in mistake-filled projects and

show up late for meetings, which prevents you from achieving the success you have always wanted.

- It is your brain that helps you devote the time to practicing so you can play the guitar like a pro, or that compels you to blow off rehearsal so you never master the instrument.

- It is your brain that controls the way you handle your money and helps you invest wisely so you can enjoy financial security or drives you to spend your paychecks before you get them so you are always in the hole.

- It is your brain that gives you the quickness and coordination to chase down shots on the tennis court so you get an athletic scholarship for college, or that makes you feel sluggish and awkward so you get picked last for team sports.

Your brain matters! The road to recovery from addiction starts with optimizing your brain. When you boost your brain, it can make it so much easier for you to gain control of your life. In the Introduction, I introduced you to the concept of addiction as an elevator that only goes in one direction: down. The only way to get off that elevator and go back up toward the life you always wanted is to take care of your brain. In this chapter, you will discover ten ways to boost your brain to get control of your life.

1. Love Your Brain

You love your vanilla latte. You love your chocolate cheesecake. You love your cigarettes. You love your bong. You love your meth. But do you love your brain? Unfortunately, most people have no love, honor, or respect for their brains. Take Judson, for example. He loved his pot. He loved his cocaine. He loved his methamphetamines. He really loved his OxyContin. By the time he was eighteen, he was hooked on drugs. He resisted going to a treatment center because he was in total denial about his addiction. His father had to drag him into the Amen Clinics against his will.

But something amazing happened when Judson looked at his brain scans. Seeing the toxic, scalloped appearance of his brain compared to the scans of healthy brains, it finally dawned on him that the drugs he was taking were seriously harming his brain, his body, and his ability to be his best self.

At that very moment, this eighteen-year-old fell in love with his brain and developed "brain envy." He wanted his brain to look like the beautiful, symmetrical, healthy brains I had shown him. He also wanted the type of life that comes with a healthy brain. And he was willing to do whatever it took to make it happen.

This young man, who had been heading downward on the addiction elevator, jumped off and started climbing his way back up. Instead of popping OxyContin pills, he started taking vitamins and supplements to support his brain health. Instead of smoking meth to feel a sensation of euphoria, he joined a gym and found that exercising gave him a mood boost. Not only that, he found that it reduced his cravings for drugs.

After six months, he landed a job in the entertainment industry, which had always been his dream. Judson's newfound love for his brain spilled over into love for the brains of those around him, and he started to worry about his girlfriend's brain. Like Judson, she had been taking all sorts of drugs for a few years, and her life was heading nowhere fast. He brought her to the Amen Clinics so she could learn to love her brain and stop doing drugs.

When you love your brain, you will find it so much easier to love your life! If you give your brain the attention it deserves, you are much more likely to gain control of your life and break free from your addictions.

2. Protect Your Brain

Your brain is very soft. Comprised of about 80 percent water, the brain's consistency can be compared to soft butter, custard, or tofu—somewhere between raw egg whites and Jell-O. To protect your soft brain, it is housed in a really hard skull filled with fluid.

Inside your skull, there are a number of bony edges and ridges. Some of these ridges are as sharp as knives and can damage your soft brain in the event of a head injury or trauma. Your brain was not meant for hitting soccer balls with your head, playing tackle football, boxing, ultimate fighting, or crashing against the concrete when you black out from being loaded.

Even mild head injuries that do not typically show up on the structural brain imaging tests can seriously impact your life and increase your risk for addiction and relapse. That is because trauma can affect not only the brain's hardware or physical health, but also its software or how it functions. Head injuries can disrupt and alter neurochemical functioning, resulting in emotional and behavioral problems, including an increased risk for relapse.

Brain trauma is much more common than you think. Each year, two million new brain injuries are reported, and millions more go unreported. People with alcohol and drug addictions are at increased risk for head injuries because they tend to do risky things like driving while drunk, plus they can lose their sense of balance because alcohol and some drugs reduce activity in the cerebellum, which is the brain's motor control center.

Take Paloma, twenty-eight, for example. She was addicted to heroin and routinely blacked out when she was partying. One morning, she woke up and discovered a huge lump on her left temple. She must have fallen and hit her head, but she had no idea how it happened. The night before was a total blank. Since that time, she has struggled with memory problems and anger issues.

For other people, there is no question what caused the brain trauma. At the Amen Clinics, we are conducting the largest brain imaging study on retired NFL players. Many of the more than ninety former professional football players we have scanned have suffered brain trauma from all those hard hits on the football field. Some of the players with the most damage have struggled with alcohol, drug, or overeating problems.

NFL Brain Damage   **Bicycle Accident**

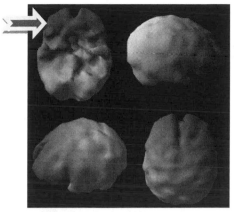   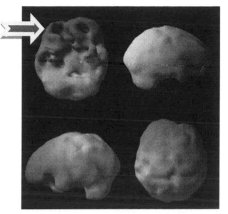

Damage to prefrontal and   *Damage to prefrontal and*
temporal lobes   *temporal lobes*

Brain injuries damage your brain and can ruin your life. They make you more vulnerable to alcoholism and drug abuse and increase your risk of relapse. Protecting your brain from injury and treating prior brain injuries gives you a better chance at recovery.

3. Feed Your Brain to Prevent Relapse

Everybody should eat a healthy diet, but as an addict you need to be especially careful about the foods you eat because they can either help your brain and keep you on track with your recovery or hurt your brain and set you up for relapse. If you have a junk-food diet, you will have a junk-food brain that is more likely to allow you to give in to your cravings. If you eat a diet filled with nutrient-rich foods, you boost your brain and your ability to say "no" to your cravings. In Chapter 11: Eat Right to Think Right and Heal from Your Addiction, you will discover the ten rules of brain healthy eating to prevent relapse.

4. Rest Your Brain

Are you getting enough sleep? Teens need nine hours of sleep at night, and adults and seniors need seven to eight hours. Getting less than six hours of sleep at night has been associated with lower overall brain activity. Research also shows that when you don't get enough sleep, you are inclined to gulp more caffeine, smoke more, exercise less, and drink more alcohol. Studies also reveal that sleep-deprived adolescents are more likely to drink alcohol, smoke marijuana, and use other drugs than young people who do get adequate sleep. Sleep-deprived people are also more inclined to skip breakfast or other meals, which puts blood sugar levels on a rollercoaster ride that's bad for brain function and often leads to poor choices later in the day, like giving in to your addiction.

Lack of sleep is also associated with weight gain and obesity. In fact, it nearly doubles the risk of obesity in adults and children. People who skimp on sleep eat an average of 221 more calories per day, tend to eat more sugary treats, and are more likely to pack on pounds than individuals who get adequate rest.

How is sleep linked to food cravings and weight? The body's appetite hormones, ghrelin and leptin, are regulated, in part, during sleep. In healthy brains, ghrelin levels rise to signal that you are hungry, then leptin levels increase to tell you when you are full. Researchers have found that lack of sleep results in higher levels of ghrelin and lower levels of leptin. This means that no matter how much you eat, you still feel hungry, causing you to overeat.

In Chapter 13: Manage Your Stress That Triggers Relapse, you will find tips to help you get more restful sleep.

5. Work Your Brain

The brain is like a muscle. The more you use it, the stronger it gets. New learning makes new connections in the brain, making you sharper and making your brain work more efficiently. No learning actually causes the brain to disconnect itself. Unlike a muscle, however, the brain gets easily bored and requires new and different challenges to maintain peak mental performance. Once the brain really learns something, such as how to play Led Zeppelin's *Stairway to Heaven* on guitar, it uses less and less energy to accomplish the task.

To keep the brain active, you need to give it a constant stream of new challenges. Acquiring new knowledge and new skills encourages brain health. Too many people, when they finish school, never think about the need to work out their brains. A healthy brain workout is not simply doing crossword puzzles. That works a specific part of your brain only. You want to work out *many* parts of your brain. Just doing word puzzles is like doing right biceps curls and nothing else, then thinking you're done with your workout.

Here are some workouts for brain specific areas.

- Prefrontal cortex
  o crossword puzzles and word games help the language areas of your brain
  o meditation boosts prefrontal function
  o hypnosis can help focus and boost prefrontal cortex function
- Temporal lobes
  o memory games
  o naming games
- Basal ganglia
  o deep relaxation
  o hand-warming techniques
  o diaphragmatic breathing
- Deep limbic
  o killing the ANTs (automatic negative thoughts)
  o gratitude practice
- Parietal lobes
  o juggling
  o interior design
- Cerebellum
  o dancing
  o table tennis (also works prefrontal cortex)
  o martial arts, without risk for brain injury ☺ (also works prefrontal cortex and temporal lobes)
  o handwriting or calligraphy

Keeping up on the latest advances in brain science can also help your brain. Signing up for our free newsletter online at www.amenclinics.com can be good for your brain. My team and I give you the latest developments in brain science and how it applies to your life. When you read the newsletter, it stretches your neurons because you're storing more information and exercising the storage and memory parts of your brain. Good brain fitness, in other words, is more akin to cross-training at the gym—exercising in a variety of ways helps improve overall performance.

Here are three more simple ways to give your brain a workout.

Break your routine. This is especially important for anyone trying to overcome addiction. You can increase your chances of recovery if you change your daily habits and routines. Introducing new habits can help rewire your brain so you don't fall back into the same patterns of activity. For example, if you always take the same route home from work and stop at your favorite bar along the way where you end up having way too many drinks, take a different route home and stop at the gym instead of hitting the bar. Eventually, you will train your brain to look forward to this new habit rather than the old destructive one.

Here are a few ideas to get you started.

- For breakfast, make a fruit smoothie instead of having coffee and a cigarette.
- Make a new friend—someone who is addiction-free and living a brain healthy life.
- Contact an old friend you haven't talked to since you became enslaved to your addiction.
- Read a book about a subject that is completely new to you.
- Listen to a different genre of music than you usually do.

Learn something new. Boost your brain by learning something new every day of your life. As little as fifteen minutes a day devoted to new learning can help optimize your brain. Here are a few examples of ways to spark better brain performance.

- Try out some new brain healthy recipes.
- Learn a foreign language.
- Take a class in something outside your major.
- Learn to play a musical instrument or a different instrument than you normally play.
- Try a sport you've never tried.
- Cross-train at work and learn how to do someone else's job.

Sharpen your skills. Although learning things that are completely new to you offer the biggest brain boost, taking your current skills to new levels by pushing yourself to improve is also beneficial. Look at the following for ideas on how to hone your skills.

- If you like to paint, try new painting techniques.
- If you play tennis, play against more talented players.
- If you like crossword puzzles, tackle more difficult ones.
- If you play guitar, try more challenging songs.
- If you knit, try more complicated patterns.

6. Exercise Your Body for Your Brain

You have probably heard the term "runner's high." Is it really possible to feel that good, just from exercise? You bet it is. Exercise can activate the same pathways in the brain as morphine and increases the release of endorphins, natural feel-good neurotransmitters. Exercise does a lot more than give you a temporary mood boost. Physical activity is the single most important thing you can do to enhance brain function. A wealth of scientific evidence shows that exercise encourages the growth of new brain cells, boosts cognitive ability in people of all ages, alleviates anxiety and depression, eases ADD symptoms, and helps prevent or delay dementia and Alzheimer's disease.

That's not all. New research shows that exercise is helpful in the prevention and treatment of addiction. Physical activity actually reduces cravings for addictive substances like cigarettes, alcohol, high-calorie foods, and drugs. It has also been shown to diminish the compulsion to gamble. In a 2006 study in *Pediatrics*, researchers found that compared to teens who watch a lot of TV, those who take part in a wide variety of physical activities are less likely to drink, smoke cigarettes, take drugs, be violent, engage in sexual activity, or partake in other forms of delinquency.

Which types of exercise are best for your brain and how much do you need to do? Doing coordination activities—like dancing, tennis, or table tennis (the world's best brain sport)—that incorporate aerobic activity and coordination are the best brain boosters. The aerobic activity spawns new brain cells while the coordination moves strengthen the connections between those new cells so your brain can recruit them for other purposes, such as thinking, learning, and remembering.

The coordination center of the brain is the cerebellum, which is linked to the PFC, where judgment and decision-making occurs. If you lack coordination, it may indicate that you are not very good at making good decisions either, making you vulnerable to addiction and relapse. Increasing coordination exercises can activate the cerebellum, thereby improving your judgment so you can make better decisions.

In general, I recommend that anybody trying to break free from an addiction do some form of aerobic coordination activity at least four to five times a week for at least thirty minutes. Some of the six types of addicts require more than that. See specific recommendations for your type on the next page.

Type 1 Compulsive Addicts. Aerobic exercise boosts serotonin in the brain to help you get unstuck when you can't stop thinking about food, cigarettes, gambling, or other addictions. Be sure to vary your workout each time. This will help you learn to be less rigid. When you get stuck on thoughts about food, alcohol, or cigarettes, get up and move! One study found that as little as five minutes of exercise could help curb cravings for cigarettes.

Type 2 Impulsive Addicts. Aerobic exercise helps increase blood flow and dopamine in the brain to boost the PFC and improve impulse control. People with this type need LOTS of aerobic exercise. At least thirty minutes a day is best, but make sure it is in an activity you love. If you don't love it, you probably won't keep it up. Also try a form of yoga that includes meditation, which will sharpen your focus and strengthen your PFC.

Type 3 Impulsive-Compulsive Addicts. Do an aerobic coordination workout for at least thirty minutes a day. Choose three activities you love, and then vary them throughout the week. Adding meditative yoga can boost your PFC and your willpower.

Type 4 Sad or Emotional Addicts. Try aerobic coordination activities that are social activities, like dancing. Or join a local tennis club or basketball team. The aerobic activity boosts blood flow and multiple neurotransmitters in the brain. The social bonding aspect of the activity can help calm the hyperactivity in the deep limbic system and enhance your mood.

Type 5 Anxious Addicts. In addition to aerobic coordination workouts, try taking yoga or t'ai chi for relaxation. Relaxation exercises can soothe overactive basal ganglia to reduce anxiety.

Type 6 Temporal Lobe Addicts. Aerobic coordination activities that involve music, such as dancing or group classes at the gym, can help boost activity in the temporal lobes.

Don't think you can just exercise your way through withdrawal and then go back to your old couch-potato ways. Several studies have found that the brain benefits of exercise are only temporary. If you stop exercising, your cravings are likely to intensify and your risk of relapse increases. Make exercise a lifelong habit, like brushing your teeth, to help you stay free of your addiction for the rest of your life.

7. De-stress Your Brain

Did you know that stress is one of the most common causes of relapse among drug abusers and smokers? Having to take a big test, getting stuck in traffic, or having an argument with a friend can be all it takes to make a recovering addict race back to heroin, painkillers, or cigarettes. It can also trigger people with other types of addictions to race for the nearest bar, Krispy Kreme, or casino. Getting a handle on stress is critical if you want to say goodbye to your addictions. Be aware that you will never be able to eliminate all the stress from your life. What you can do is learn better coping skills. In Chapter 13: Manage Your Stress That Triggers Relapse, you will find many healthy ways to deal with stress so you can stay on track with your recovery.

8. Kill the ANTs That Infest Your Brain

One of my favorite people in our retired NFL players study, Big Ed White from the Minnesota Vikings, weighed 365 pounds when I first met him. When I asked him about his weight, he told me that he had no control over his eating. That was his automatic response.

"I have no control."

"Is that true?" I asked. "You really have NO control over your eating?"

He paused and said, "No. That really isn't true. I do have some control."

"You know," I told him, "just by thinking that you have no control, you have just given yourself permission to eat anything you want at any time you want."

Big Ed White was infested with ANTs. ANTs stands for automatic negative thoughts, the thoughts that come into your mind and ruin your day. Most people think of being overweight as an eating disorder, which is certainly true, but it is also a thinking disorder! All addictions for that matter are thinking disorders.

Believing the lies that you tell yourself, like "It's your fault that I drink so much," "I can't go to a party without snorting cocaine or

170

I'll be boring and nobody will like me," or "I only smoke so I won't gain weight" keeps you in chains. To break free, you need to learn to challenge these thoughts. In Chapter 14: Kill the Addiction ANTs That Infest Your Brain and Keep You in Chains, you will learn how to talk back to your thoughts so you can get control of your thinking and your life.

9. Serenade Your Brain

Do you remember the song you first slow danced to? The song that played at your wedding? The song you were listening to when your first boyfriend or girlfriend broke up with you? Most people do. Music is the soundtrack of our lives. It moves us emotionally and can lift our mood when we're feeling blue, calm our nerves when we're feeling anxious, or pump us up before a big game. Certain kinds of music also make us feel angry, lonely, or depressed. We all know this instinctually, but there's also science to back it up.

For decades, neuroscientists have been uncovering the ways that listening to and playing music changes our brains… for the better. Music is so powerful, it can actually help your efforts to become addiction-free. This is especially true for Type 6 Temporal Lobe Addicts because the temporal lobes are heavily involved in processing music. Here are some of the ways you can use music to boost your brain so you can stay on track with healthier habits.

Sing. Singing stimulates temporal lobe function, which is involved with memory and learning, so it is very beneficial for Type 6 Temporal Lobe Addicts. Singing expands the lungs and pumps up the flow of oxygen to the brain, which boosts brain function. Singing in the morning helps wake you up, stimulates the rhythms of life, boosts your mood (especially helpful for Type 4 Sad or Emotional Addicts), and makes you more mentally alert for the day's activities. No wonder so many of us like singing in the shower! Don't restrict your singing to the shower though. Sing whenever and wherever you can for better brain function. Humming can also improve mood and memory.

Learn to play a musical instrument. It's never too late, or too

171

early, to learn to play a musical instrument. A tremendous amount of scientific research shows that music lessons boost IQ, enhance memory, and improve emotional health. In young people, it has been found to increase test scores and improve achievement in math.

Learning how to strum a guitar or tinkle the ivories requires the orchestration of many areas of the brain, including the frontal lobes (attention, planning, follow-through), parietal lobes (direction sense, sense of touch, seeing objects in space), temporal lobes (memory, reading, and language), coordination centers (cerebellum), emotional centers (mood control, motivation, attitude), and sensory systems (touch, sight, sound). By learning to read music, you also stimulate the brain's visual cortex (sight). Because music training integrates nearly all the senses and involves almost every known cognitive process, it is one of the best brain-boosting activities you can try.

Listen to your iPod. We all know that music can make us feel better, and there's scientific evidence to prove it. Studies have shown that listening to and playing music can decrease depression, reduce anxiety and stress, lower blood pressure, maintain cognitive function in the elderly, lower heart rate, relieve pain, improve sleep, and increase focus in children with ADD. Type 4 Sad or Emotional Addicts should listen to bright happy tunes that lift your mood. Type 5 Anxious Addicts can benefit from soothing music and nature sounds.

Move with music. When we listen to or play music, we often can't help but tap our feet, bob our heads, or sing along. Music also encourages us to engage in more complex movements, such as dancing to a waltz or trying to keep up with the music on the video game Dance Dance Revolution. Making love with music in the background represents a passionate combination of the way music moves us both emotionally and physically. Moving physically with music activates the coordination centers of the brain. Considering the coordination centers are linked to the decision-making, judgment, and impulse control centers, music may be able to improve your self-control.

10. Treat any Brain Problems Early

Mental (brain) health illnesses, such as ADD, depression, bipolar disorder, anxiety disorders, obsessive-compulsive disorders, schizophrenia, grief, and posttraumatic stress disorder all take a very real toll on you. These disorders are intensely stressful, rob you of sleep, alter your appetite, and increase your risk for relapse. It is essential to treat these brain health problems as early as possible so they do not become a stumbling block to your recovery. Be aware though that the highs and lows associated with substance abuse can mimic the symptoms of brain disorders, and you may need to wait until you have gone through withdrawal to determine if you really have a mental health issue.

Bad Brain Habits Quiz

Do you have too many bad brain habits? Answer the following questions to find out if your daily habits are harming your brain. You can also find these questions in the Unchain Your Brain Master Questionnaire in Appendix A.

Please rate each question on a scale of 0–4.

0 = Never	3 = Frequently
1 = Rarely	4 = Very frequently
2 = Occasionally	N/A = Not applicable

_____ 1. My diet is poor and tends to be haphazard.

_____ 2. I do not exercise.

_____ 3. I put myself at risk for brain injuries by doing such things as not wearing my seat belt, drinking and driving, engaging in high-risk sports, etc.

_____ 4. I live under daily or chronic stress in my home or work life.

_____ 5. My thoughts tend to be negative, worried, or angry.

_____ 6. I have problems getting at least seven to eight hours of sleep a night.

_____ 7. I smoke or am exposed to secondhand smoke.

_____ 8. I drink or consume more than two normal-size cups of coffee, tea, or dark sodas a day.

_____ 9. I use aspartame and/or MSG.

_____ 10. I am around environmental toxins, such as paint fumes, hair or nail salon fumes, or pesticides.

_____ 11. I spend more than one hour a day watching TV.

_____ 12. I spend more than one hour a day playing computer or video games.

_____ 13. Outside of work time, I spend more than one hour a day on the computer.

_____ 14. I have more than three normal-size drinks of alcohol a week.

_____ 15. I tend to eat too much.

_____ 16. I skip meals.

_____ 17. I tend to eat a lot of high-fat, high-sugar snacks like cookies and cakes or refined carbohydrates like muffins, bagels, and scones.

_____ 18. I am constantly checking my email, Facebook, or Twitter accounts.

Your Score:
0–6   Great brain habits; keep it up.
7–12   Really good; work to be better.
13–20   Fair; you are prematurely aging your brain.
>20   Poor; time to be very concerned.

UNCHAIN YOUR BRAIN CHECKLIST

✓ Develop brain envy.

✓ Protect your brain from injury to prevent relapse.

✓ Eat brain healthy foods to boost your brain and willpower.

✓ Get at least seven hours of sleep, at least nine hours if you are a teenager.

✓ Learn something new every day.

✓ Get a minimum of thirty minutes of exercise at least four to five times a week.

✓ Choose physical activities that are best for your brain type.

✓ Learn how to deal with daily stress.

✓ Talk back to your ANTs.

✓ Sing, play a musical instrument, and listen to music geared to your type.

✓ Don't wait to treat brain problems.

Chapter 10

Step #5

CRAVING CONTROL

Nine Ways to Lock Up the Craving Monster That Steals Your Life

Cravings never go away. You just have to learn to outsmart them.

Trevor, thirty-nine, was doing really well in a twenty-eight-day treatment program for cocaine addiction. By the time he reached graduation day, he thought he had kicked the habit and would never again be a slave to the drug. But then he went home, and reality hit. When he went to work the following week, he was so swamped with a backlog of work that he skipped lunch in favor of a bag of chips from the vending machine. Taking his normal route to the vending machine, he had to pass by the sales department, where he crossed paths with Brandon, one of his cocaine buddies from that department. Just seeing Brandon triggered memories of using, and all of a sudden, the old familiar cravings crept back into his brain.

He was so unnerved by the incident and so starving that he headed back to the vending machine that afternoon and bought two candy bars and a diet soda to try to deal with the cravings. That night when Trevor got home, he was so irritated and stressed out about his day that he lashed out at his wife when she greeted him. It turned into a big fight, and he stormed out of the house. His cravings were so intense that he headed straight to his cocaine supplier and got high. All of the hard work he had put into getting clean deteriorated rapidly.

What went wrong? Trevor didn't want to use again, but he couldn't control his cravings. Could Trevor have done anything differently so he would have had a better chance or preventing the relapse? Definitely! Now let's replay Trevor's day with a few tweaks to show how he could have gotten better control of his cravings.

When Trevor went back to work after his stint in a treatment facility, he set up a meeting with his supervisor to talk about how to handle his workload. Together, they devised a plan so Trevor could enlist the help of a few of his colleagues to plow through the stacks on his desk. He knew he would be very busy at work so he had prepared a sack lunch that morning consisting of a spinach salad with salmon, blueberries, walnuts, avocado, and a little olive oil and lemon. At lunchtime, he sat at his desk and ate the salad while he worked. Thanks to the good nutrition, he was able to think clearly during the afternoon.

When he wanted an afternoon snack, he thought about how hard it would be for him to pass by the sales department and his cocaine buddies who work there, so he took a different route to the vending machine where he bought an apple. By the time he got home that night, he was feeling pretty good about the progress he had made at work and the fact that he had made it through another day without using cocaine. He greeted his wife with a hug and a kiss. They had dinner together and mapped out a strategy for dealing with the following day's potential cravings.

Like Trevor, you can make simple changes to your daily habits in order to get better control of your cravings. But don't expect your cravings to go away... EVER. In Chapter 4: How Addictions Get Stuck in Your Brain And How to Get Them Unstuck, you learned about the brain's reward system and how it hijacks your brain so your cravings take control of your life. You also need to understand that once you have crossed the line into addiction, you have effectively rewired your brain to make it more susceptible to those intense cravings, for the rest of your life.

Depending on what you are addicted to, just seeing a glass pipe used for smoking cocaine, smelling cookies baking in the food court at the mall, or talking to your drinking buddy will spark the emotional memory centers in your brain and trigger your cravings. Even after decades of sobriety or steering clear of gambling, bulimia, or Internet porn, your brain is still vulnerable to cravings.

Take my patient Molly, for example. At age fifty-eight, after thirty-two years of staying clean from heroin addiction, Molly had to have a surgical procedure. The doctor prescribed Vicodin—an opiate like heroin—for post-surgical pain relief. When Molly took one, it fired up those old addicted pathways in her brain and ratcheted up cravings for the drug she had quit taking so many years before.

Fortunately, Molly had anticipated this could be a problem, and she had given the bottle of Vicodin to her husband and put him in charge of hiding them from her, counting them out each day, and dispensing them to her as directed on the bottle. After a couple of days, her pain was more bearable, and she switched to non-opiate, over-the-counter pain relievers, and the cravings subsided.

Because you are so vulnerable to cravings, it is critical to learn how to keep them at bay. In this chapter, I will give you nine essential strategies to get control of your cravings so you can avoid relapse.

1. Keep Your Blood Sugar Balanced

Low blood sugar levels are associated with lower overall brain activity, including lower activity in the PFC, the brain's brake. Low brain activity here means more cravings and more bad decisions. As mentioned before, in a 2007 article, Matthew Gailliot and Roy Baumeister detailed the connection between blood sugar levels and self-control. They write that self-control failures are more likely to occur when blood sugar is low. Low blood sugar levels can make you feel hungry, irritable, or anxious—all of which make you more likely to make poor choices.

What causes low blood sugar levels? Many everyday behaviors can cause dips in blood sugar levels, including drinking alcohol, skipping meals, and consuming sugary snacks or beverages. High-sugar treats and drinks actually cause an initial spike in blood sugar, but then a crash about thirty minutes later. Gailliot and Baumeister's study also indicates that the body uses glucose less efficiently as the day progresses, leading to more self-control failures in the evening and later at night.

Here are five tips to keep your blood sugar levels even throughout the day so you can reduce cravings and boost your self-control.

Consider taking the supplements alpha-lipoic acid and chromium. They both have very good scientific evidence that they help balance blood sugar levels and can help with cravings. Find more on these supplements later in this chapter.

Eat a nutritious breakfast every day. Eating a nutrient-rich breakfast helps get your blood sugar get off to a good start and can help keep it balanced for hours so you don't get hungry before lunchtime. Studies show that people who maintain weight loss eat a healthy breakfast. Find out what types of foods to eat in Chapter 11: Eat Right to Think Right and Heal from Your Addiction.

Have smaller meals throughout the day. This helps eliminate the blood sugar rollercoaster ride that can impact your emotions and increase your cravings.

Stay away from simple sugars and refined carbohydrates. This includes candy, sodas, cookies, crackers, white rice, white bread, and sweetened juices. High-sugar, high-fat foods work on the addiction centers of the brain. This is critical for people who are addicted to overeating, and for people with other types of addictions. Bingeing on sugar has been found to alter brain chemistry and raise the risk for indulging in drugs or alcohol.

In fact, sugar addiction is common in alcoholics and often develops when alcoholics try to quit drinking. Because alcohol is metabolized in the body the same way sugar is, eating sugar can fuel alcohol cravings, and vice versa. Professor Bart Hoebel and a team of researchers from Princeton University have been studying sugar addiction in rats for several years. In one of their trials, they found that when sugar-addicted rats were deprived of sucrose, they started drinking more alcohol than normal. Similarly, rats that consumed more alcohol increased intake of sugar.

> **Hoebel and his colleagues suggest that
> sugar addiction can be a "gateway" to other addictions.**

If overeating is a problem for you, you definitely have to avoid the dessert table. When I finally got this one idea through my own thick skull it made a huge difference for me, and I was finally able to lose the extra pounds I had been trying to shed for years. I love living without cravings. But, for years I fought the idea of giving up sweets, like Rocky Road ice cream or candy. I thought the key to losing weight was simply about calories in versus calories out. If I stayed within a certain calorie range I would be fine. The problem was that eating the sugar activated my cravings and made it very hard to stay away from things that were bad for me.

Sweets are mood foods for me. My grandfather was a candy maker and my best memories growing up were standing at the stove next to him making fudge or pralines. But my grandfather was also overweight and had two heart attacks that took him away from me way too early. I know that kicking the sugar habit isn't easy for many people—it is like kicking a drug—and it certainly wasn't easy for me, but I found that when I substituted brain healthy fruit like blueberries, bananas, and apples, the cravings completely went away. Have you ever known someone to eat too many blueberries? For most people, it takes about two weeks of completely avoiding sugar for your dessert cravings to go away.

2. Decrease the Artificial Sweeteners

If you really want to decrease your cravings, you have to get rid of the artificial sweeteners in your diet. We think of these sweeteners as free, because they have no calories, but because they are up to six hundred times sweeter than sugar, they may activate the appetite centers of the brain making you crave even more food and more sugar. A group of Australian scientists found that alcohol

180

floods the bloodstream faster when it is mixed with beverages containing artificial sweeteners rather than sugar. Diet sodas are NOT the answer. The one "natural" no-calorie sweetener I like is called stevia.

3. Manage Your Stress

Another very important way to decrease your cravings is to get on a daily stress-management program. Anything stressful can trigger certain hormones that activate your cravings, making you believe that you NEED the ice cream, cigarettes, or cocaine. Meditation and hypnosis are wonderful stress-management practices that can help boost your brain so you can get control of your cravings. I will talk about these more in Chapter 13: Manage Your Stress That Triggers Relapse.

4. Outsmart Sneaky Addiction Triggers

To control your cravings you also have to outsmart the sneaky triggers that try to sabotage you nearly everywhere you go. For Trevor, the simple act of walking down the hall at work and seeing his cocaine buddy sparked cravings for the drug. No matter what you are addicted to, there are environmental triggers all around. If you are an alcoholic, driving past your favorite bar or walking down the liquor aisle in the grocery store can fuel your desire to drink again. If cigarettes are your drug of choice, and you go to a party where someone is smoking, the smell of it can ignite your brain's emotional memory centers and make you feel like you HAVE to have a cigarette.

If you're an overeater, you can't go to the mall, the airport, or the ball game without seeing store after store and vendor after vendor advertising something that will fire up your cravings. For example, whenever I went to the movies, I used to immediately think about getting a BIG tub of popcorn with lots of butter along with licorice. But then I actually thought about the gobs of saturated fat, salt, and sugar that would be flooding my brain. Another trigger for me is going over to my mom's house on holidays—she makes the most amazing pizzas. I could easily eat eight slices, but end up feeling stuffed and stupid.

To control your cravings, you have to control your triggers. Know the people, places, and things that fuel your cravings and plan ahead for your vulnerable times. For example, I take a snack with me when I go to the movies now so I am not tempted by the popcorn and licorice, and I eat a little something ahead of time before going over to my mom's house on holidays, so that my brain can choose to eat a slice or two of pizza without blowing the whole holiday season in one thirty-minute gorge.

5. Find Out About Hidden Food Allergies

Hidden food allergies and food sensitivities can trigger cravings and make you relapse. For example, did you know that wheat gluten and milk allergies can decrease blood flow to the brain and decrease your judgment? In addition, many of the symptoms associated with food allergies, such as headaches, sleep problems, lack of concentration, and anxiety, can increase stress and cravings.

Food allergies are closely linked to alcoholism. Corn, wheat, rye, and barley are common sources of food allergies and also happen to be ingredients used to make alcohol like vodka, whiskey, beer, gin, and bourbon. Remember that the foods you are allergic to are often the ones you crave the most, so if you are allergic to an ingredient in alcohol, you may crave alcohol.

See Chapter 7: Getting the Right Evaluation for more on food allergies and how to get tested for them.

6. Practice Willpower to Retrain Your Brain

Willpower is like a muscle. You have to use it or lose it. Most of us learn to develop self-control as children. When our parents say "no" to us when we ask if we can do things that aren't good for us—have a plate of cookies before dinner, ride on the back of a neighbor's motorcycle without a helmet, or grab the tail of a strange dog—we learn to say "no" to ourselves. But maybe your parents weren't around much, and you had free rein to do whatever you wanted so you never learned self-control. Or perhaps your parents had addictions, and you learned to give in to your desires by watching their behavior. Or perhaps your addiction has robbed you of your ability to say "no."

No matter what the reason is for your lack of willpower, you can strengthen it. To pump up your willpower, you need to practice it. Make it a habit to say "no" to the things that are not good for you and over time, you will find it easier to do.

Long-term potentiation (LTP) is a very important concept here. When nerve cell connections become strengthened, they are said to be potentiated. Whenever we learn something new, our brains make new connections. At first the connections are weak, which is why we do not remember new things unless we practice them over time. Practicing a behavior, such as saying "no" to meth, alcohol, doughnuts, or gambling, actually strengthens the willpower circuits in the brain. LTP occurs when nerve cell circuits are strengthened, practiced, and behaviors become almost automatic. Whenever you give in to your addiction it weakens your willpower and makes it more likely you will continue to give in. When you practice willpower, your brain will make it easier for you.

7. Get Moving

In Chapter 9: Boost Your Brain to Get Control, you discovered why exercise is so important for a better brain. Scientific research on exercise and addiction has found that physical activity can cut cravings and reduce the risk for relapse. Whether you crave cigarettes, alcohol, sugary snacks, drugs, or gambling, exercise can help. One study of moderately heavy smokers who had abstained from smoking for fifteen hours showed that even when faced with smoking-related images that would typically trigger cravings, the smokers had less desire to light up after exercising.

A 2007 study in the journal *Addiction* showed that cravings for cigarettes decrease rapidly during exercise and remain diminished for up to fifty minutes after physical activity. In this trial, it didn't matter whether participants did high-intensity exercise for thirty to forty minutes or short bouts of low-intensity activity. Any amount of activity, even as little as five minutes, helped tone down cravings. This is important to remember when cravings hit. Instead of giving in or focusing on how much you want something, get moving if at all possible.

8. Get Adequate Sleep

Have you ever noticed that after a night with almost no sleep, you wake up ravenously hungry and want to eat anything and everything in sight? That is because lack of sleep increases food cravings, as I described in Chapter 9: Boost Your Brain to Get Control. It also increases cravings for other addictive behaviors. Find out how to get more restful sleep so you can minimize those urges in Chapter 13: Manage Your Stress That Triggers Relapse.

9. Take Natural Supplements for Craving Control

N-acetyl-cysteine, alpha-lipoic acid, chromium, dl-phenylalanine, and l-glutamine are five amazing natural supplements that can help take the edge off cravings. Here's how they work.

N-acetyl-cysteine (NAC): NAC is an amino acid that is needed to produce glutathione, a very powerful antioxidant. NAC binds to and removes dangerous toxic elements within the cells, making it a molecule critical to brain health. Recently, NAC has been studied as a treatment for drug addiction, as it functions to restore levels of the excitatory neurotransmitter glutamate in the reward center of the brain. A growing body of research has found that NAC can reduce cravings for cocaine, heroin, and cigarettes and decrease the risk for relapse. It also reduces compulsive behavior in pathological gamblers and may be helpful in reducing food cravings.

One of the key findings in several studies on NAC and cocaine is that the supplement helps reverse the neurobiological changes that occur with addiction and make users more vulnerable to relapse. Other research concludes that NAC shows promise for the treatment of compulsive behavior problems. This means it could be helpful for Type 1 Compulsive Addicts who are addicted to gambling, overeating, or sex, as well as those with impulsive-compulsive eating disorders, such as bulimia.

In one study, researchers in the Department of Psychiatry at the University of Minnesota conducted a double-blind, placebo-controlled clinical trial on NAC and its effects on twenty-seven pathological gamblers. After the eight-week trial, 83 percent of those taking NAC compared to only 29 percent of placebo-takers experienced at least a 30 percent reduction in addictive behavior. The typical adult dose is 600 to 1,200 mg twice a day to curb cravings.

Alpha-lipoic acid: Made naturally in the body, alpha-lipoic acid may protect against cell damage in a variety of conditions. There is strong evidence that alpha-lipoic acid supports stable blood sugar levels. Studies have shown that it improves insulin sensitivity and may be effective in treating type 2 diabetes. The typical recommended adult dose is 100 mg twice a day.

Chromium: Chromium picolinate is a nutritional supplement used to aid the body in the regulation of insulin, which enhances its ability to efficiently metabolize glucose and fat. There is a strong link between depression, decreased insulin sensitivity, and diabetes. Supplementation with chromium picolinate has been shown to effectively modulate carbohydrate cravings and appetite, which is beneficial to managing both the diabetes and depression.

I often recommend chromium picolinate to help with insulin regulation and to control carb cravings. In a well-designed study, 600 micrograms of chromium picolinate was beneficial for patients with atypical depression (the type of depression where people gain weight, rather than lose weight), especially those with carbohydrate cravings. Scientists at Oxford University in England demonstrated with animals that supplementing the diet with chromium enhances the activity of neurochemicals associated with mood control within the brain.

It is believed that chromium may help raise serotonin levels by facilitating the transport of certain amino acids within the brain and central nervous system. This could explain why it is helpful in reducing cravings for refined carbohydrates, which also raise serotonin levels. The typical recommended adult dosage is 200 to 600 micrograms a day.

DL-phenylalanine: This is an essential amino acid (cannot be produced by the body) and thus must be obtained through the diet. Phenylalanine is used in different biochemical processes to produce the neurotransmitters dopamine, norepinephrine, and epinephrine. There is evidence that phenylalanine can increase mental alertness, release hormones affecting appetite, and reduce drug and alcohol cravings.

There have been reports that L-phenylalanine can promote high blood pressure in those predisposed to hypertension. Monitoring in the first few months on phenylalanine can detect blood pressure increases in the minority of people who will have this symptom. Phenylalanine can promote the cell division of existing malignant melanoma cells. If you have melanoma, or any other form of cancer for that matter, avoid phenylalanine. Persons who have PKU (phenylketonuria) cannot use phenylalanine. This includes those born with a genetic deficiency that prevents them from metabolizing phenylalanine. The typical recommended starting dosage for adults is 500 mg a day, and slowly work up to 1,500 mg a day.

L-glutamine: L-glutamine is an amino acid that is important in the synthesis of the excitatory neurotransmitter glutamate and the inhibitor neurotransmitter GABA. It is also a nutrient for the brain as it is used for energy if the brain does not have enough glucose to function. Supplemental glutamine has been used in the treatment of ADD, anxiety, and depression. It has been shown to decrease carbohydrate cravings. The typical adult dose is 500 mg three to four times a day.

Dr. Daniel Amen's Nutraceutical Solutions: Craving Control

Given what I know about craving and nutritional supplements, I developed a special formula to help support craving control. You can learn more about it at www.amenclinics.com. As we have seen, the key to controlling your cravings is balancing your brain and maintaining healthy blood sugar levels. In support of this goal, Craving Control supports healthy blood sugar levels while providing antioxidants and brain healthy nutrients. The formulation includes glutamine to reduce cravings, chromium and alpha-lipoic acid to support stable blood sugar levels and a brain-healthy chocolate designed to boost endorphins. In addition, the super-antioxidant N-acetyl-cysteine is added, which has been shown in clinical studies to reduce cravings in a number of different conditions.

UNCHAIN YOUR BRAIN CHECKLIST

- ✓ Keep your blood sugar balanced.

- ✓ Decrease the artificial sweeteners.

- ✓ Manage your stress.

- ✓ Outsmart sneaky addiction triggers.

- ✓ Find out about hidden food allergies.

- ✓ Practice willpower to retrain your brain.

- ✓ Get moving.

- ✓ Get adequate sleep.

- ✓ Take natural supplements for craving control.

Chapter 11

Step #6

EAT RIGHT TO THINK RIGHT

And Heal From Your Addiction
Junk-food diet = junk-food brain.

Melinda, twenty-nine, was always worried about gaining weight. During the day, she would take speed and drink lots of caffeine to suppress her appetite. For breakfast, she would have a large Frappa-something loaded with artificial sweeteners and nonfat milk to cut the calories. Lunch consisted of a few bites of French fries from the local fast-food joint followed by more coffee and handfuls of candy that she kept in her desk at work. Dinner was usually a slice of pizza. At night, she liked going out with her friends to get buzzed. When she went to bars, she was afraid of getting fat from the high-calorie cocktails, so instead of having ten drinks, she would limit herself to four drinks and then pop a few Valium to get the high she was looking for.

When Melinda decided that she needed help getting off the drugs and alcohol, she joined a support group. At the meetings, they served coffee and doughnuts, and Melinda helped herself to several cups of coffee and at least a few doughnuts. At home and work, she started drinking even more coffee and eating more candy. She also started ordering hamburgers for lunch in addition to her French fries and eating several slices of pizza for dinner. Three months after Melinda had kicked her drug and alcohol habits, she had gained twelve pounds and felt terrible all day long. She had headaches, fatigue, fuzzy thinking, irritability, and moodiness. Plus, her cravings for coffee and candy had skyrocketed and her cravings for speed, alcohol, and Valium weren't going away. If this was what being sober was like,

188

Melinda didn't like it! Every day was a battle to stay clean, and after four months, she couldn't resist and relapsed.

Melinda made a common mistake that many people in recovery make—eating all the wrong things. A junk-food diet can put you on the fast track to relapse, whether you are addicted to drugs and alcohol, gambling, or Internet porn. Changing your relationship with food is critical to your success, and this doesn't apply only to people with eating disorders, such as bulimia, anorexia, or overeating. If you want to break free from addiction, you have to understand that food isn't just something to binge on; it's something that should nurture your brain and body so you can have the life you always wanted.

Take seventeen-year-old Siobhan, for example. When she entered a treatment program for drug and alcohol addiction, her diet consisted of doughnuts, fast food, candy, and diet sodas. Working in the organic garden on the facility's premises and helping cook meals using the herbs and vegetables she had helped grow slowly started to change her perspective about food. She no longer thought of it as a "quick fix" to feed her emotional troubles or to get a sugar rush. Instead, she began to see that by nourishing the garden with water, mulch, and love, she was creating foods that would in turn nourish her brain and body. This new relationship with food helped her overcome her addictions.

Beware: if you are taking part in a support group or treatment program for your addiction, don't expect that the food being served is the best for your brain or your recovery. Some programs and groups do a great job of providing nutritious foods, but others get an F in the nutrition department. I have found that in some treatment facilities, patients can wander the halls and buy cookies, candy, or Coke from vending machines. And in many group meetings, like the ones Melinda attended, foods and beverages that are counterproductive to recovery are readily available. You have to take charge of what you put in your body.

In this chapter, you will find the Amen Clinics ten rules for brain healthy nutrition to prevent relapse. Note that I call them "rules" because people who have addictions typically don't have a strong self-control circuit or a healthy internal brake. Because of this, you need external rules to help guide you to do the right things. When it's a rule, you have to follow it, no questions asked.

Rule #1: Think High-Quality Calories In Versus High-Quality Energy Out

Don't let anyone tell you that calories don't count. They absolutely do. But maintaining a healthy weight and eating right is not as simple as calories in versus calories out. I want you to think about eating mostly high-quality calories. One cinnamon roll can cost you 720 calories, will drain your brain, and will increase your cravings. A 400-calorie salad made of spinach, salmon, blueberries, apples, walnuts, and red bell peppers will supercharge your energy and help you think more clearly so you can make better decisions throughout the day.

The research about calories is very clear. If you eat more calories than you need, you will be fatter, sicker, and less productive. In the famous rhesus monkey study, researchers followed a large group of monkeys for twenty years. One group ate all the food they wanted; the other group ate 30 percent less. The monkeys who ate anything they wanted were three times more likely to suffer from cancer, heart disease, and diabetes. Plus researchers saw significant shrinkage in the important decision-making areas of their brains.

Chronic overeating reduces your ability to make the right choices, increasing your risk for relapse. Eating a little bit less than you need helps keep your brain functioning optimally. But don't go overboard and starve yourself. Lack of nutrients deprives the brain of the fuel it needs and leads to dysfunction and possible relapse.

University of Wisconsin
Rhesus Monkey Calorie-Restriction Study

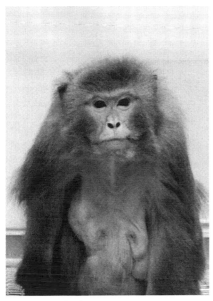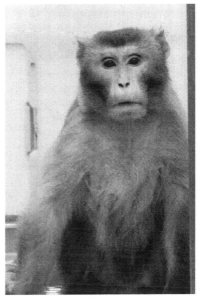

No Restrictions   Ate 30 Percent Less

Images used with permission of Jeff Miller, Senior Photographer at the University of Wisconsin

You need to know how many calories a day you need to achieve or maintain a healthy weight. You can find calculators on the Amen Clinics website (www.amenclinics.com/cybcyb) that tell you how many calories you need based on your current or goal weight, gender, age, and activity level. The average active fifty-year-old man needs about 2,200 calories a day to maintain his weight, and most adult women need about 1,800 calories. To lose a pound a week, you have to eat 500 fewer calories a day than you need.

You also need to know how many calories a day you actually put in your body, just like you need to know how much money you spend. Overeating is the exact same thing as overspending. When you overeat, you bankrupt your brain and body. Similarly, severely undereating robs strength from your brain and body. If weight is a problem for you, keep a daily food journal just like you keep a checkbook. Start the day with the number of calories you can spend, and write down everything you eat or drink. This will give you a sense of where you are throughout the day.

This one strategy made a huge difference for me. When I actually wrote down everything I ate for a month, it caused me to stop lying to myself about my calories. One of the men in our retired NFL players study wrote that when he started counting his calories, it opened a new world of self-abuse that he was completely unaware of. Keeping a food journal can be a real eye-opener. On the Amen Clinics website, there is a great journal to help you get started.

What about the second part of this rule? By high-quality energy out, I mean exercise. That is the healthiest way to work off the calories you consume. Trying to reduce your caloric intake with diet pills or loads of caffeine, or getting rid of calories with laxatives or purging is detrimental to your health and recovery.

Rule #2: Drink Plenty of Water and Not Too Many of Your Calories

Your brain is 80 percent water. Anything that dehydrates it, such as too much caffeine or much alcohol, decreases your thinking and impairs your judgment. Make sure you get plenty of water every day. I recommend drinking half your weight in ounces in water. For example, if you weigh 180 pounds, you should be drinking 90 ounces of water.

On a trip to New York City recently I saw a poster that read, "Are You Pouring On The Pounds… Don't Drink Yourself Fat." I thought it was brilliant. A recent study found that on average, Americans drink 450 calories a day, twice as many as we did thirty years ago. Just adding the extra 225 calories a day will add twenty-three pounds of fat a year to your body, and people tend to NOT count the calories they drink. Did you know that some coffee drinks or some cocktails, such as margaritas, can cost you more than 700 calories each? And they provide absolutely nothing in the way of nutrients.

In fact, most calorie-laden beverages—sodas, coffee drinks, alcohol, and energy drinks—contain ingredients that decrease brain function and set you up for relapse. Of course, if you are addicted to alcohol, you shouldn't be drinking alcoholic beverages. Avoiding alcohol is important for all types of addicts because beer, wine, and liquor impair your judgment and thinking.

One very simple strategy that can not only help you lose a lot of weight but also improve brain performance is to eliminate most of the calories you drink. My favorite drink is water mixed with a little lemon juice and a little bit of the natural sweetener stevia. It tastes like lemonade, so I feel like I'm spoiling myself, and it has virtually no calories.

Rule #3: Eat High-Quality Lean Protein throughout the Day

Protein helps balance your blood sugar and provides the necessary building blocks for brain health. Eating protein is important for people with all types of addictions, but it is critical for Type 2 Impulsive Addicts. Higher-protein diets tend to help this type focus and stay on track.

Protein contains L-tyrosine, an amino acid that that is important in the synthesis of brain neurotransmitters. Found in foods like meat, poultry, fish, and tofu, it is the precursor to dopamine, epinephrine, and norepinephrine, which are critical for balancing mood and energy. It is also helpful in the process of producing thyroid hormones, which are important in metabolism and energy production. Tyrosine supplementation has been shown to improve cognitive performance under periods of stress and fatigue. Stress tends to deplete the neurotransmitter norepinephrine, and tyrosine is the amino acid building block to replenish it.

Also found in protein is L-tryptophan, an amino acid building block for serotonin. L-tryptophan is found in meat, eggs, and milk.

Increasing intake of L-tryptophan is very helpful for some people in stabilizing mood, improving mental clarity and sleep, and decreasing aggressiveness. Scientific evidence also shows that supplementation with L-tryptophan can help people lose weight.

Eating protein-rich foods like fish, chicken, and beef also provides the amino acid glutamine, which serves as the precursor to the neurotransmitter GABA. GABA is reported in the herbal literature to work in much the same way as antianxiety drugs and anticonvulsants. It helps stabilize nerve cells by decreasing their tendency to fire erratically or excessively. This means it has a calming effect for people who struggle with temper, irritability, and anxiety, whether these symptoms relate to anxiety or temporal lobe disturbance.

Great sources of lean protein include fish, skinless turkey or chicken, beans, raw nuts, and high-protein vegetables, such as broccoli and spinach. Did you know that spinach is nearly 50 percent protein? I use it instead of lettuce on my sandwiches for a huge nutrition boost.

Rule #4: Eat Low-Glycemic, High-Fiber Carbohydrates

This means eat carbohydrates that do not spike your blood sugar and that are also high in fiber, such as whole grains, vegetables, and fruits like blueberries and apples. Carbohydrates are not the enemy. They are essential to your life. Bad carbohydrates are the enemy. These are carbohydrates that have been robbed of any nutritional value, such as simple sugars and refined carbohydrates. If you want to live without cravings, eliminate these completely from your diet. I like the old saying, "the whiter the bread the faster you are dead."

Sugar is not your friend. Sugar increases inflammation in your body and increases erratic brain cell firing. Plus, new research shows that sugar is addictive and can even be more addictive than cocaine. Here is an example of extreme sugar addiction. I saw a feature on ESPN about Los Angeles Lakers forward Lamar Odom, who has a terrible sweet tooth, consuming up to 80 dollars worth of candy a week. As a Lakers season ticket holder, I have suffered through years of Odom's erratic on-court performances. I decided to write a piece for my blog, which was picked up by the *Los Angeles Times*, which subsequently, caused a firestorm of controversy during the 2009 NBA finals. Here is an excerpt of the piece.

The Lakers' Lamar Odom, Sweet Tooth, and Erratic Play

I have been a huge Los Angeles Lakers fan since I was a child. I am really excited about my team being in the NBA Finals for the second year in a row. What I'm not as excited about is a piece I recently watched on ESPN about Lakers star Lamar Odom and his massive addiction... to candy. In it, you can see the 6-foot 10-inch forward gobbling up massive quantities of the sugary treats.

Odom has been a giant source of frustration for Lakers fans. He is unbelievably talented, but often acts like a space cadet during games. Once, he was taking the ball out on the sidelines, when he walked onto the court before he threw the ball in, causing a turnover. During the Lakers last home game against the Denver Nuggets, Kobe Bryant threw him a pass, but the ball hit him on the shoulder because he had spaced out and was not paying attention. On talk shows, Odom is constantly criticized because no one knows if he will play well or not. He can play great, and be worth his fourteen-million-dollar a year salary or he can act like he is "missing in action."

Odom freely confesses that he just can't help himself when it comes to the sweet stuff and always keeps a stash on hand of Gummi Bears, Honey Buns, Lifesavers, Hershey's Cookies 'n' Crème white chocolate bars, Snickers bars, cookies, and more. He eats the sugary snacks morning noon and night, and even says he sometimes wakes up in the middle of the night, chows down on some treats, then falls back asleep.

This is bad news for the Lakers. I've been telling my patients for decades that sugar acts like a drug in the brain. It causes blood sugar levels to spike and then crash, leaving you feeling tired, irritable, foggy, and stupid. Eating too much sugar impairs cognitive function, which may explain why Odom doesn't always make the smartest decisions on the court.

Excessive sugar consumption also promotes inflammation, which can make your joints ache, and delay healing from injuries, which is definitely a bad thing for a professional athlete. It is also linked to headaches, mood swings, and weight gain. Weight gain isn't a problem now for Odom, but it is for the average person who isn't playing full-court basketball for hours each day.

As a fan and a physician, it concerns me that our professional sports organizations and players are not more concerned about brain health, which includes nutrition. My advice to Odom and to all sugar addicts is to get your sugar consumption under control. You will feel so much better and your brain will function better, too.

After my piece ran, I was interviewed by ESPN radio and reporters played part of my interview for Odom. Odom, like most addicts, denied it was a problem, and said he had eaten candy for breakfast during games five, six, and seven of the last round of the playoffs against the Denver Nuggets, and he had played well in those games. The problem with the comment, however, was that there was no game seven. The Lakers won it in six games. Lakers' coach Phil Jackson was also asked about my comments and said he knows candy makes kids more troubled and when you have kids, "Halloween is the worst night of the year." If Odom wants to be a world-class athlete who performs consistently, he needs to eat a brain-healthy diet. If you want to break free from addiction, you do, too.

Sugar addiction is also associated with other addictions so you have to be careful with it. My co-author David is a prime example. Ever since he quit drinking and smoking pot, he has had a problem with sweets. "I can't eat any sugar—zippo," he says. "If I have one bite of sugar, something happens in my brain, and I want to wipe out the whole plate."

A lot of people ask me, "Isn't it okay to have sweets in moderation?" Personally, I don't agree with the people who say, "Everything in moderation." Cocaine or arsenic in moderation is not a good idea. Sugar in moderation triggers cravings. The less sugar in your life the better your life will be. Reach for a banana or an apple instead.

Rule #5: Focus Your Diet on Healthy Fats

If you want to prevent relapse, increase your intake of omega-3 fatty acids. These are healthy fats that come from foods like wild salmon, tuna, mackerel, avocados, walnuts, and olive oil. Low levels of omega-3 fatty acids have been associated with depression, anxiety, obesity, and ADD. There is also scientific evidence that low levels of omega-3 fatty acids play a role in substance abuse and risk for relapse.

According to a 2003 study in *Psychiatry Research*, low levels of omega-3 fatty acids increased the risk for relapse in cocaine addicts. For this study, researchers analyzed omega-3 levels of thirty-eight cocaine addicts shortly after admission to a treatment program. They followed up with the participants by retesting omega-3 levels and assessing relapse status at intervals of three, six and twelve months following discharge. Subjects who relapsed at three months had significantly lower baseline omega-3 levels compared to people who had not relapsed. The lower baseline omega-3 levels were also associated with higher levels of relapse at six and twelve months following discharge from the treatment program.

Eliminate bad fats, such as ALL trans-fats and most animal fat from your diet. Did you know that fat stores toxic materials? So when you eat animal fat, you are also eating anything toxic the animal ate. Yuk. Here's something that is especially important for people who are addicted to overeating. Did you know that certain fats that are found in pizza, ice cream, and cheeseburgers fool the brain into ignoring the signals that you should be full? No wonder I used to always eat two bowls of ice cream and eight slices of pizza!

High cholesterol levels are not good for your brain. A new study reports that people who have high cholesterol levels in their forties have a higher risk of getting Alzheimer's disease in their sixties and seventies. The B vitamin niacin has very good scientific evidence it helps lower cholesterol. Avocados and garlic can help as well. A little guacamole anyone? But don't let your cholesterol levels go too low. Did you know that low cholesterol levels have been associated with both homicide and suicide? If I am at a party and someone is bragging to me about their low cholesterol levels, I am always VERY nice to that person.

Rule #6: Eat From the Rainbow

Put natural foods in your diet of many different colors, such as blueberries, pomegranates, yellow squash, and red bell peppers. This will boost the antioxidant levels in your body and help keep your brain young. This does not mean Skittles or jelly beans.

Rule #7: Cook with Brain Healthy Herbs and Spices to Boost Your Brain

Here is a little food for thought, literally. The herbs and spices in your kitchen cupboards can give your brain the boost it needs. Ounce for ounce, herbs and spices pack more antioxidant punch than most fruits and vegetables and provide powerful protection for that three-pound supercomputer between your ears.

198

Here are some of the most potent brain spices:

- Turmeric, found in curry, contains a chemical that has been shown to decrease the plaques in the brain thought to be responsible for Alzheimer's disease.
- In four studies, a saffron extract was found to be as effective as antidepressant medication in treating people with major depression.
- Sage has very good scientific evidence that it helps to boost memory.
- Cinnamon has been shown to help attention. Plus, cinnamon is a natural aphrodisiac for men. My wife makes an amazing sweet potato soup with slivered almonds, cranberries, cinnamon, and sage. It makes me smarter and more affectionate at the same time.

Rule #8: Limit Caffeine

When you are trying to break free from your addictions, you must steer clear of caffeinated coffee, tea, sodas, chocolate, energy drinks, and diet pills. Caffeine is a stimulant that can trigger cravings for other addictive drugs and behaviors. Excessive consumption can also lead to caffeine addiction, which comes with its own set of withdrawal symptoms, including headaches, irritability, fatigue, and low moods.

If you have a problem with caffeine addiction and you want to kick the habit, do it gradually. Taper off your intake over several weeks to minimize withdrawal symptoms. If caffeine isn't your problem, don't let it become one! Far too many addicts simply trade one addiction for another. For example, many alcoholics and drug addicts turn to caffeine to help them cope with the way they feel during the withdrawal and recovery process, but then they get addicted to the caffeine buzz.

Here are some of the many ways that caffeine harms the brain and increases your risk for relapse.

- Caffeine restricts blood flow to the brain, which leads to impaired judgment and more bad decisions.
- Caffeine dehydrates the brain and lowers overall function.
- Caffeine interferes with sleep, which wreaks havoc with your energy, moods, and thinking.
- Caffeine can increase anxiety, which raises stress levels.

Rule #9: Take a Daily Multiple Vitamin, Fish Oil, and Natural Supplements for Your Brain Type

People with active addictions usually have diets that are devoid of brain healthy nutrients. Ninety-one percent of Americans do not eat at least five servings of fruits and vegetables a day, the minimum required to get good nutrition. For years, I have been advocating that everybody take a daily multivitamin. The American Medical Association (AMA) agrees. For twenty-two years, the AMA recommended against taking a daily multivitamin, but reversed its position. The AMA now recommends daily vitamins for everybody because they help prevent chronic illness.

Taking vitamins is critical for people with all types of addictions because it can help restore the brain and body to health. A lot of people argue that if you are eating a balanced diet, you don't need a supplement. That may be true, but how many addicts do you know who are eating a perfectly nutritious diet every day?

In addition to a daily multiple vitamin/mineral supplement, I almost always prescribe a fish oil supplement for patients dealing with addictions, regardless of their brain type. Fish oil is a great source for omega-3 fatty acids, which you learned about in Rule #5 above. Fish oil is important for everybody, but it is even more critical for recovering alcoholics and drug addicts.

Here's why. In the above Rule #3, you learned how L-tyrosine, which is found in protein, is involved in the production of dopamine. In healthy people, enzymes convert L-tyrosine into dopamine, which can improve moods and emotions as well as attention span and the ability to think clearly. In people with drug and alcohol addictions, however, the enzymes don't work as efficiently so the L-tyrosine being consumed in protein may not get converted into dopamine. That can be a stumbling point for people in recovery and can exacerbate mood and emotional issues, lack of attention, and fuzzy thinking—all of which can raise the risk for relapse. Taking fish oil supplements has been found to improve enzyme efficiency so L-tyrosine can be converted to dopamine.

Depending on your brain type, you may benefit from other natural supplements. See Chapter 8: Know Your Brain Type for more specific details on types and supplements.

Rule #10: Eat Right for Less

Addiction can be very costly in so many ways and people often find themselves in dire financial straits as a result. Fortunately, you don't have to spend a bundle to eat right. I recently wrote a blog on brain healthy eating for the poor. In writing the blog, I asked for some help from my esteemed friend Dr. Jeff Fortuna, the author of *Nutrition for the Focused Brain* and *Food, Brain Chemistry and Behavior*. Dr. Fortuna is a faculty member in the Department of Health Science at California State University, Fullerton, and the clinical nutritionist for Newport Academy, a residential treatment program for teens suffering from drug abuse and co-occurring disorders. Together, we came up with the following ten tips to help people eat healthier without spending a fortune.

Go for satisfying grains. When it comes to grains, you can't beat old-fashioned oatmeal or pearled barley, which cost about 10 cents or less per serving. These bargain whole grains offer a huge nutritional bang for your buck, moderate blood sugar for hours, and keep you feeling full longer.

Buy vitamin-rich vegetables frozen and save. Stock up on frozen vegetables like broccoli, spinach, and carrots whenever you go to a warehouse store like Costco. It's cheaper than buying fresh and can cost you as little as 11 cents a serving.

Boost antioxidants with apples, oranges, and bananas. Affordable apples and oranges (less than 50 cents each) and bananas (less than 20 cents each) are full of vitamins and antioxidants that promote health and boost brain performance.

Say cheese—cottage cheese, that is. Cottage cheese is packed with protein, calcium, and vitamins A and D. With a single serving of cottage cheese, you get 13 grams of protein for about 75 cents. Just make sure you are one of the lucky ones who process dairy. Being lactose intolerant can drop blood flow to the brain and make you more impulsive.

Pump up protein with affordable eggs. Getting adequate amounts of protein doesn't have to involve eating expensive meat. At less than 20 cents apiece, protein-rich eggs are an affordable option for breakfast, lunch, or dinner.

Fill up on high-fiber, low-cost beans. Loaded with fiber and high in protein, beans should be a staple in any household that is struggling financially. For example, a 1-pound bag of black beans costs less than $2, and gives you twelve servings for less than 16 cents each.

Stock up on canned tuna. Eating fish like tuna is a great source of omega-3 fatty acids. You can get a three-pack of tuna for about $2.50, which means for about 83 cents a can, you get 22 grams of protein and a good amount of healthy omega-3 fatty acids. Be careful not to overdo the tuna as it may contain some mercury.

Drink to your brain health with skim milk and water. Low in fat and high in protein and calcium, skim milk is fortified with vitamins A and D and will only set you back about 25 cents for one serving. You don't need to buy pricey bottled water. With a $15-$20 water filter that fits on your kitchen faucet, you can drink from the tap and get healthy, filtered water that will keep your brain and body hydrated for optimal performance.

Spice up your meals. With just a few spices in your cupboard, you can enhance the flavor of any dish without using a lot of unhealthy butter, cream, or salt. You can find spices for a few dollars each—they're even cheaper if you can buy them loose where you scoop the spices into bags rather than buying them in a bottle.

Become a savvy shopper. You can save a bundle if you buy items that have a long shelf life—like canned tuna, beans, oatmeal, barley, and frozen vegetables—in bulk. Look for sales and specials, use coupons, and buy generic brands when possible. You can even shop online for many food items or look for coupons online from local stores to find the best deals.

UNCHAIN YOUR BRAIN CHECKLIST

- ✓ Watch your calories.

- ✓ Choose water over other beverages.

- ✓ Make lean protein part of every meal.

- ✓ Eat more vegetables and fruits.

- ✓ Get more omega-3 fatty acids in your diet.

- ✓ Eat a variety of colorful fruits and vegetables.

- ✓ Use brain-boosting spices and herbs to add flavor rather than calorie-laden cream sauces or butter.

- ✓ Cut the caffeine.

- ✓ Take a multi-vitamin, fish oil, and other natural supplements for your brain type.

- ✓ Be a smart shopper and save.

Chapter 12

Step #7

KILL THE ANTS THAT INFEST YOUR BRAIN

And Keep You in Chains

You don't have to believe every stupid thought you have.

M ost people plagued with addictions are filled with what we call ANTs or automatic negative thoughts; negative thoughts that come into their minds automatically, drive their addictions, and ruin their days. They focus on the bad things that have happened or the frightening things that may happen and subsequently make themselves sick and more vulnerable to give in to their negative behaviors.

"I have no control over my eating… drinking… smoking."

"I only smoke pot because you make me so miserable."

"My dad was an alcoholic so I'm destined to be one too."

"I only bet on sports with my friends, so I don't have a gambling problem."

"I am so awful, no one will love or forgive me."

"I smoke so I can spend time with other smokers I like."

"My mother smoked and ate poorly and lived well into her nineties. I have great genes."

You do not have to believe every thought you have. Thoughts lie. They lie a lot, and these lies can fool you, scare you, tease you, and ruin your life. Learning how to kill the ANTs and develop an internal ANTeater to help you get rid of the negative thoughts has been shown in scientific studies to be as effective as antidepressant medications to treat anxiety and depression and can help you unchain your brain.

Addiction Isn't Just a Brain Disorder; It's a Thinking Disorder

Many of the negative things we tell ourselves—like *"I have no control"*—are lies that keep us locked in our unhealthy ways. In the addiction field, these lies are often referred to as "stinking thinking" or "white-knuckle sobriety." There's a common saying among addiction experts: *"Relapse is a process, not just an event, and it's predated by stinking thinking."*

I think of these negative thoughts like ANTs that infest your psyche and keep you in chains. Your thoughts are powerful. Bad, mad, sad, hopeless, or helpless thoughts release chemicals that make you feel bad and increase your risk of relapse.

In this chapter, you will learn how to develop an internal ANTeater to patrol the streets of your mind and talk back to the lies you tell yourself. This method of challenging your thoughts to help prevent relapse is backed by strong scientific evidence. A 2009 review of fifty-three controlled trials using this method concluded that it is an effective strategy for treating substance abuse. You will also discover how to turn negative thinking into healthy, honest thinking. Did you know that happy, positive, hopeful, loving thoughts release chemicals that make you feel good? Honest thinking can help you feel better and keep you away from the buffet, coffee pot, bars, casinos, video games, cigarettes, or drugs.

Nine ANTs That Keep You in Chains

Over the years therapists have identified nine "species" of ANTs or types of negative thoughts that can increase your risk for relapse:

1. All or nothing
2. Always thinking
3. Focusing on the negative
4. Thinking with your feelings
5. Guilt beating
6. Labeling
7. Fortune telling
8. Mind reading
9. Blame and denial

1. All or nothing

One obese player in our retired NFL players study told me that he was fat because he just didn't like any of the foods that were healthy for him. "Is that really true?" I asked. "You don't like ANY of them?" I then showed him a list of our fifty best brain healthy foods, and in fact, he liked about 60 percent of them. This is an example of all or nothing thinking, when you believe that everything is all good or all bad. It is the same as black-or-white thinking. Here are a couple more examples:

"I am seven days clean, I have got this licked."

"I just relapsed. I am the worst alcoholic on the planet."

"We had an argument. I think it's over."

"I didn't do well on the test. I'm a terrible student and should just quit college."

If you stick to your brain healthy eating plan for a month, you think you are the most disciplined person on the planet. If you stop for fast food one day because you didn't have time for breakfast and you're starving, you think you have no discipline, give up on your new eating habits, and go back to eating junk food on a daily basis. Everybody runs into speed bumps and small failures in life, but that doesn't mean that YOU are a failure. A better approach is to acknowledge that you ate food that wasn't the best for your brain or your recovery and then get back on track the following day. One slip-up doesn't mean you should give up entirely.

2. Always thinking

This is when you overgeneralize a situation. Always thinking usually involves words, such as always, never, every time, or everyone. Here are some examples:

"I will never be able to stop smoking."

"I have always been fat; it will never change."

"Every time I get stressed, I have to have a drink."

This kind of thinking sentences you to a lifetime of addiction. It makes you believe you have no control over your actions and behaviors and that you are incapable of changing them.

3. Focusing on the negative

So many addicts focus on the negative and ignore the positive side of situations. This ANT can take a positive experience, work interactions, or relationships, and taint it with negativity. It is the judge, jury, and executioner of new relationships and new habits.

"I got together with an old friend who doesn't use drugs, but she showed up ten minutes late for lunch, so I'm not going to call her again."

"I went to the gym and did a hard workout, but the guy on the bike next to me was talking the whole time, so I'm never going back there."

"I cut back my caffeine intake from ten cups of coffee a day to two, but I wanted to get down to no coffee by now, so I should just quit trying."

Focusing on the negative makes you feel bad, and that increases your chances for relapse. It can also make you more inclined to give up on your efforts to lead a brain healthy life. Try focusing on the positive and it will improve your mood and make you feel better about yourself. Putting a positive spin on your thoughts leads to positive changes in your brain. Here's how you could think about these same situations:

"I met up with an old friend, and it felt really nice to reconnect with someone outside of my circle of drug-using friends."

"After working out, I had a lot more energy for the rest of the day."

"Wow! I'm down to drinking only two cups of coffee a day. I'm doing so much better than before and am on my way to my goal of eliminating it completely."

4. Thinking with your feelings

These ANTs occur when you have a feeling about something, and you assume it is correct so you never question it. Feelings can lie, too. These thoughts usually begin with the words "I feel."

"I feel stupid."

"I feel like a loser."

"I feel like you don't love me anymore."

"I feel like nobody will ever trust me."

"I feel like you're mad at me."

Whenever you have a strong negative feeling, check it out. Look for the evidence behind the feeling. Do you have real reasons to feel that way? Or, are you feelings based on events or things from the past?

5. Guilt beating

Guilt is generally not a helpful emotion. In fact, guilt often causes you to do those things that you don't want to do. Thinking in words like "should," "must," "ought to," and "have to" are typical with this ANT. Here are some examples:

"I should have stopped by now."

"I have to get to the meeting or I will relapse."

"I ought to spend more time with my family"

The problem is that when we feel pushed or guilted into doing things, our natural tendency is to push back. It is better to replace "guilt beatings" with phrases like "I want to do this," "It fits with my goals to do that," or "It would be helpful to do this." In the examples above, it would be beneficial to change the phrases to:

"It is my goal to stop doing my negative behaviors because my health, job, and family are important to me."

"I want to get to the meeting because it will be useful to my sobriety."

"It is in my best interest to spend time with my family because I love them and want to protect our relationships."

6. Labeling

When you call yourself or someone else names or use negative terms to describe them, you have a labeling ANT in your brain. A lot of us do this on a regular basis. You may have said one of the following at some point in your life:

"He's a jerk."

"She's lazy."

"I'm a loser."

"He's a drunk."

"I'm a druggie."

The problem with negative labels is they exercise negative pathways in the brain and make them stronger. Negative pathways can lead to negative behaviors. Calling yourself names is very detrimental to the recovery process because it takes away your control over your actions and behaviors. For example, if you are a "loser," then why bother trying to change your behaviors? It is as if you have given up before you have even tried. This defeatist attitude can keep you enslaved to addiction.

When you "label" others you also lump them with all the other people in your memory bank to whom you gave a similar label and cannot deal with them any more on an individual or rational basis. For example, if, in your head, you say someone is a drunk then you lump them with all the drunks you have ever known and cannot see them as an individual person.

Beware Of The Red Ants

These last four ANTs are the worst. I call them the red ANTs because they can really sting and increase your risk for relapse.

7. Fortune telling

Predicting the worst even though you don't know what will happen is the hallmark of the fortune telling ANT. You probably have these ANTs in your brain if you've ever said anything like:

"When football season comes around, I know I won't be able to avoid gambling."

"If I try to eat a healthy diet, I know I'll cheat."

"I know I'm going to relapse."

The problem with fortune telling is that your mind is so powerful that it can make happen what you see. So when you are convinced that you are going to relapse, you don't try as hard to overcome your addiction, and you increase your odds of falling back into your old habits.

Nobody is safe from fortune telling ANTs, not even me. Several years ago, I wrote an article for *Parade* magazine called "How to Get Out of Your Own Way." After the article was published, my office received more than ten thousand letters asking for more information about self-defeating behavior. The media got wind of the response, and I was invited to appear on CNN. It was a great opportunity for me to get the word out about the work we do here at the Amen Clinics, but I had never been on TV before, and I was nervous—*really* nervous.

I was sitting in the "green room" right before I went on and all of a sudden, I had a panic attack. I couldn't breathe, my heart was racing, and I wanted to get the heck out of there. Thankfully, I treat people with this problem. I told myself the same things I tell my patients:

"If you are having a panic attack in a safe situation, don't leave or panic will rule your life. Slow down your breathing. Write down your thoughts and what kind of ANTs they are."

So I stayed put, took a deep breath, and grabbed a pen to write down my thoughts.

"I'm going to forget my name"—fortune telling.

"I'm going to stutter"—fortune telling.

"Two million people are going to think I'm stupid"—fortune telling.

With just one look, I knew that I had a fortune telling ANT infestation. Then, just like I tell my patients, I told myself to talk back to my thoughts.

"Okay, if I forget my name, I have my driver's license in my pocket and can look it up."

"I don't usually stutter, but if I do, all the stutterers out there watching will have a doctor they can relate to."

And as for people thinking I'm stupid, I reminded myself of the 18/40/60 rule, which says when you are eighteen you worry about what everybody is thinking of you. At forty you don't give a damn what anyone else thinks. And, at sixty, you realize that nobody has been thinking about you at all. Most people spend their days worrying and thinking about themselves.

This little exercise helped calm me down so I was able to go on TV, and I did fine. I did not forget my name. I did not stutter. And I did not get phone calls, letters, or emails from two million people telling me I was stupid. The next time I was asked to appear on TV, I was not quite as nervous. And with each subsequent appearance, I became more relaxed. Since that first time, I have appeared on TV more than one hundred times, and it no longer makes me nervous at all. Just think if I had listened to my lying, fortune telling ANTs and had run out of the studio. I probably never would have accepted another invitation to be on TV, and it would have dramatically changed my life and career in a negative way.

8. Mind reading

When you think you know what others are thinking even though they have not told you, and you have not asked them, it is called mind reading. Mind reading is a common cause of trouble between people. It frequently happens in intimate relationships because one partner assumes they can read the other's mind. It doesn't work because you can never know what others are thinking. You are probably familiar with these mind-reading ANTs:

"He doesn't like me."

"They were talking about me."

"They think I will never amount to much."

I have twenty-five years of education—mostly in how to diagnose, treat, and help people—and I can't read anyone's mind. I have no idea what they are thinking unless they tell me. A glance in your direction doesn't mean somebody is talking about you or mad at you. I tell people that a negative look from someone else may be nothing more than his being constipated! You just don't know. When there are things you don't understand, ask for clarification, and stay away from mind reading ANTs. They are very infectious and cause trouble between people.

9. Blame and denial (the most dangerous Red ANTs)

Of all the ANTs, the blame and denial ANT is the one that really hurts. Blame and denial are very harmful. Blaming others for your problems is toxic thinking. When you blame something or someone else for the problems in your life, you become a victim of circumstances and you cannot do anything to change your situation. You know the kind of thoughts I'm talking about:

"I wouldn't have gotten a DUI if we had taken the other street like I wanted to instead of going your way."

"It's not my fault I eat too much; my mom taught me to clean my plate."

"I only started smoking because you smoke, so it's your fault I can't quit."

Here's an extreme example of how blaming others can keep you in chains. Stephen, twenty-seven, was addicted to meth. While using a blowtorch to light the meth, he managed to set fire to his house. Later, he sued the manufacturers of the blowtorch, claiming they were to blame for the accident. When David met with Stephen, he tried to get him to see the truth by explaining the situation this way, "No meth, no blowtorch. No blowtorch, no fire." But Stephen still didn't get it. He had convinced himself that meth had absolutely nothing to do with the fire; it was all the blowtorch's fault. Stephen was in complete denial that he had a problem and that his behavior was the real reason for the fire. The legal system was an accomplice in his flawed thinking and reinforced his denial.

Here's another example. One of the players in our retired NFL players study told me that he was fat because everyone in his family was overweight. It was just his genetics. "Is that true?" I asked. "This really doesn't have anything to do with how much you eat? Your genes are not your destiny. My genes too say I am supposed to be fat." He paused, looked at me, and said, "That's a pretty lame excuse, isn't it?"

Whenever you begin a sentence with "It is your fault that I..." it can ruin your life. These ANTs make you a victim. And when you are a victim, you are powerless to change your behavior. In order to break free from addiction, you have to change your behavior, so kill the blame and denial ANTs.

Develop an Internal ANTeater to Challenge Your Erroneous Thoughts

You do not have to believe every stupid thought that goes through your brain. Develop an internal ANTeater that can kill all the negative thoughts that come into your head and mess up your life. Teach your ANTeater to talk back to the ANTs so you can free yourself from negative thinking patterns. Whenever you feel sad, mad, nervous, obsessive, or out of control, write down the automatic thoughts that are going through your mind. The act of writing them down helps to get them out of your head. Identify the ANT species then talk back to them. Challenging negative thoughts takes away their power and gives you control over your thoughts, moods, and behaviors.

214

ANT-Killing Examples

ANT	Species of ANT	Kill the ANT
You never listen to me.	Always thinking	I get frustrated when you don't listen to me, but I know you have listened to me and will again.
I'll pass out if I have to speak at my support group.	Fortune telling	I don't know that. Odds are I will do fine.
I'm unlovable.	Labeling	Sometimes I do things that push others away, but I also do many loving things.
It's your fault I have these problems.	Blame and denial	I need to look at my part of the problems and look for ways I can make the situation better.

My ANTeater Chart
Whenever you feel sad, mad, nervous, obsessive, or out of control, use the following chart to write out your thoughts and talk back to them.

ANT	Species	ANTeater
_____	_____	_____
_____	_____	_____
_____	_____	_____
_____	_____	_____

Do The Work

One of my favorite books, *Loving What Is*, comes from my friend Byron Katie. In this very wise book, Katie, as her friends call her, describes an amazing transformation that took place in her own life. At the age of forty-three, Katie, who had spent the previous ten years of her life in a downward spiral of rage, addiction, despair, and suicidal depression, woke up one morning on the floor of a halfway house to discover that all those horrible emotions were gone. In their place were feelings of utter joy and happiness.

Katie's great revelation, which came in 1986, was that it is not life that makes us feel depressed, angry, abandoned, and despairing, rather it is our thoughts that make us feel that way. This insight led Katie to the notion that our thoughts could just as easily make us feel happy, calm, connected, and joyful.

It also led her to realize that our minds and our thoughts affect our bodies. "The body is never our problem. Our problem is always a thought that we innocently believe," she wrote in her book *On Health, Sickness, and Death.* In the same book, she also wrote, "Bodies don't crave, bodies don't want, bodies don't know, don't care, don't get hungry or thirsty. It is what that mind attaches—ice cream, alcohol, drugs, sex, money—that the body reflects. There are no physical addictions, only mental ones. Body follows mind. It doesn't have a choice."

Katie wanted to share her revelation with others to help them end their suffering by changing their thinking. She developed a simple method of inquiry called The Work to question our thoughts. The Work is simple. It consists of writing down any bothersome, worrisome, or negative thoughts, then asking ourselves four questions, and then doing a turnaround. The goal of the Work isn't pie-in-the-sky positive thinking; it is honest thinking. The four questions are:

1. Is it true? (Is the negative thought true?)

2. Can I absolutely know that it is true?

3. How do I react when I think that thought?

4. Who would I be without the thought? Or how would I feel if I didn't have the thought?

After you answer the four questions, you take your original thought and turn it around to its opposite, and ask yourself whether the opposite of the original thought is true. Then, turn the original thought around and apply it to yourself (how does the opposite of the thought apply to me personally?). Then, turn the thought around to the other person if the thought involves another person (how does the opposite apply to the other person?).

I have done The Work myself many, many times, and it helped me get through a very painful period of grief. When I did The Work, I immediately felt better. I was more relaxed, less anxious, and more honest in dealing with my own thoughts and emotions. Now, I always carry the four questions with me, and I use them a lot in my practice and with my friends and family. Here is an example of how to use the four questions to kill the ANTs that are keeping you in chains.

Corinne, fifty-two, had smoked since she was a teenager. She had now smoked for almost forty years and had wrinkled skin and trouble breathing. The people who loved her wanted her to stop. She wanted to stop but didn't believe she could without serious pain. "I cannot stop," she told me. Here is how she worked on that thought.

Negative Thought: "I cannot stop smoking."

Question #1: Is it true that you cannot stop smoking?

"Yes," she said.

Question #2: Can you absolutely know that it is true that you cannot stop smoking?

Initially she said yes, she knew she couldn't do it. Then she thought about it and said, "Of course, I cannot know for sure, especially if I got the right help."

Question #3: How do you feel when you have the thought "I cannot stop smoking."

"I feel powerless, sad, weak-willed, stupid, out of control, like a bad influence on my children."

Question #4: Who would you be without the thought "I cannot stop smoking."

She thought about it for a moment then said, "Hopeful, optimistic, more likely to give it my best effort."

Turnaround: What is the opposite thought of "I cannot stop smoking." Is it true or truer than the original thought?

Corinne said the opposite thought is "I can stop smoking." She thought about this for a while and said that if she got help and really tried, it could be true. Then she felt a sense of control and committed to the program. Your thoughts are either helping you or hurting you.

As I was writing this book, I was on a tour for my public television show, "Change Your Brain, Change Your Body." On these tours I often visit up to fifteen public television stations in two weeks. Even though they are a grind, I love visiting stations to help them raise money and support my shows.

During a recent visit I was working with one of my favorite co-hosts who was on a medical weight loss plan where he was getting daily injections of pregnancy hormone while only eating 500 calories a day. I am not fond of these diets because they do not teach you how to live a brain healthy life. They are a quick fix. As we were talking during a break he told me that his diet ended at the end of that week. He said that while on the diet, because it was so restrictive, thinking about food was his new porn. He had been on it eight weeks and had lost nearly twenty pounds. He whispered to me that he had already called a famous pizza place in Chicago and had ordered two large deep-dish pizzas that he was going to devour over the weekend. He would be good starting on Monday.

"Are you serious?" I asked him in disbelief. "What about all the effort to lose the twenty pounds?"

"It is just one weekend of debauchery," he replied innocently.

My thought, that my prefrontal cortex inhibited me from actually saying, was that his recent quick-fix effort was weight loss for dummies. The lie he was telling himself was that he could cheat and it would all be okay. After all, it was just two pizzas.

As we have seen with addicts of all types, one drink or two famous deep-dish pizzas can start the addiction all over again. It is the lies you tell yourself that keep you in chains.

UNCHAIN YOUR BRAIN CHECKLIST

- ✓ Stop lying to yourself.

- ✓ Don't believe every stupid thought that goes through your brain.

- ✓ Become familiar with the nine ANTs that steal your happiness and keep you in chains.

- ✓ Develop an internal ANTeater that can talk back to your negative thoughts.

- ✓ Do The Work to challenge and eliminate negative, addiction-causing thoughts.

Chapter 13

Step #8

MANAGE YOUR STRESS THAT TRIGGERS RELAPSE

Stress is normal. The way you've been dealing with it isn't.

Most people think of stress as bad. Actually, stress is good and bad. Stress is good because it causes us to pay attention to what is going on around us—in traffic, with our finances, at work, and in our relationships. When we say something is stressful, it usually means that we should be paying attention to it. Stress is bad when it overloads our resources. Stress can motivate us (to study for an exam or pay our bills on time), it can protect us (we buy alarm systems for our homes, businesses, or cars), and it can feed us (we go to work to put food on the table).

However, too much stress can also kill you. Chronic stress has been implicated in addictions, anxiety and depressive disorders, obesity, Alzheimer's disease, heart disease, and a host of immune disorders, including cancer. When stress hits, there are increased levels of adrenaline (leading to anxiety) and cortisol (leading to many illnesses) and decreased levels of the hormones DHEA and testosterone (leading to loss of muscle tissue, increased fat, and decreased libido). Both adrenaline and cortisol are released by the adrenal glands, on top of the kidneys, in response to real or perceived stress.

The human brain is so advanced that even imagining stressful events will cause the body to react to the perceived threat as if it is actually happening. We can literally scare our body into a stress response. The brain is a powerful organ.

Adrenaline and cortisol help us deal with acute stress by

increasing energy when we are faced with a threat. They are the primary chemicals of the fight-or-flight response. Whenever there is an immediate perceived threat, such as seeing a rattlesnake in your front yard (which happened to me not too long ago), the body prepares to either run away or fight the threat. The hypothalamus in the deep emotional brain releases a chemical called CRH (corticitropin releasing hormone), which in turn stimulates the pituitary gland to produce ACTH (adrenocorticotropin hormone), which in turn stimulates the adrenal glands to produce cortisol and adrenaline.

Together these chemicals prepare the body to fight or flee. Among other things, adrenaline dilates our pupils, increasing visual acuity; shunts blood from our hands and gut to the large arm and leg muscles (so we can fight or run); increases our breathing rate and heart rate to increase oxygen to the body; and increases sweat gland activity to keep us cool. Cortisol stimulates the release of glucose, fats, and amino acids into the bloodstream for energy.

The problem with stress in our modern-day world is not these short bursts of adrenaline and cortisol. We need those reactions to deal with our rattlesnake encounters. The problem with the stress reaction is that for many of us it never stops—traffic, bills, bosses, employees, unhappy in-laws, too little sleep, illnesses, and too much to do. Chronic exposure to adrenaline causes our systems to be overloaded with too much stimulation and leads to anxiety and depression, obesity, and memory problems. Chronic exposure to cortisol can make us fat and stupid.

In normal amounts, both of these chemicals are essential. Cortisol, for example, has an initial anti-inflammatory effect (doctors use cortisol like medications to help with asthma, arthritis, colitis, and to relieve certain skin disorders). It also calms immune response in organ transplantations. In appropriate amounts, both chemicals help the body maintain internal balance.

Low levels of cortisol are associated with Addison's disease, an illness where stress can cause a dangerous drop in blood pressure and even circulatory collapse. President John F. Kennedy had Addison's disease and had to take cortisol tablets when he was under great periods of stress, such as the Cuban Missile Crisis. High levels of cortisol are related to an illness called Cushing's disease, where people have an accumulation of central body fat (making them look apple-shaped) and muscle wasting of the limbs (skinny arms and legs). Cushing's disease can be associated with immune system problems, psychotic depression, and many other health issues.

Cortisol levels can be elevated by chronic stress, addictions, intense exercise, pregnancy, depression, anxiety, and by the intake of stimulants such as ephedra or caffeine (as little as two or three cups a day). When Marine recruits are exposed to high levels of stress, such as extreme sleep deprivation or intellectual or physical stress, they have increased cortisol blood levels and decreased performance. It has also been shown that extreme endurance athletes have increased cortisol levels as well as decreased testosterone levels leading to reduced sperm counts and reduced libido. Excess in any form is stressful.

Chronic exposure to high levels of cortisol has been associated with myriad problems that make us unhappy, such as increased appetite, sugar and fat cravings, and abdominal obesity. Cortisol signals fat cells to hold onto their fat stores, leading to a high waist-to-hip ratio (WHR—the circumference of the waist divided by that of the hips), which makes you look like an apple. A person's WHR is associated with perceived attractiveness. An optimal WHR is 0.8, anything above that puts a person at risk for the illnesses mentioned above associated with higher cortisol levels. A WHR ratio of 0.7 has been associated with the most attractive women, in part because it is a sign of health and potential fertility. As we age, our figures go from being an hourglass to a shot glass (especially if we are drinking too much alcohol or eating too much sugar).

Long-term exposure to high levels of cortisol has also been associated with low energy, poor concentration, elevated cholesterol levels, heart disease, and hypertension, as well as an increased risk for strokes, diabetes (reduced sensitivity to insulin), muscle wasting, osteoporosis, anxiety, depression, irregular menstrual periods, lowered libido, and decreased fertility. High cortisol levels decrease immune system function, shrinking the thymus gland and impairing white blood cell function (as much as 50 percent following a severe stress). Chronic stress dramatically increases the use of medical services and health care costs. Stress not only increases cortisol, it decreases key anabolic hormones, such as DHEA, growth hormone, and testosterone. This combination causes you to store fat, lose muscle, slow metabolic rate, and increase your appetite.

In the last decade there has been a clear association between chronic stress, high cortisol levels, and memory problems, causing shrinkage of cells in the hippocampus of the brain. In fact, people with Alzheimer's disease have higher cortisol levels than normal aging people.

Relaxation Techniques

While the stress response puts your body on high alert, the relaxation response does the opposite. It reduces the release of stress hormone and increases the release of endorphins, the body's natural pain-killing substances. This slows your breathing rate and heart rate, reduces blood pressure, and relaxes muscles. In other words, the relaxation response is your rest and reset mode, the time when the body and mind get a chance to heal.

First documented by Harvard cardiologist Herbert Benson, the relaxation response is created when the "thinking" part of the brain "tells" the amygdala and hippocampus—in the "emotional" limbic system—to relax. The amygdala and hippocampus then relay the message to the hypothalamus, which begins orchestrating the release of a flood of calming neurotransmitters and hormones. Soon the body and brain shift into a soothing state of relaxation.

You can learn to take your body from a high-stress state to a more relaxed state by using the following techniques. These strategies can help all types of addicts, but they are especially beneficial for Type 5 Anxious Addicts who have a tendency to feel nervous, worried, or "on edge."

Deep breathing. As part of the body's natural stress response, your breathing becomes more shallow. When you take shallow breaths, it reduces the amount of oxygen that reaches your brain cells, reducing overall brain function. The simple act of breathing also serves to eliminate waste products, such as carbon dioxide, from the body, and shallow breathing can lead to a buildup of carbon dioxide. When there is too much carbon dioxide in your system, it can cause stressful feelings of disorientation and panic, things that can lead to cravings and relapse.

Deep breathing, also known as diaphragmatic breathing, is a relaxation technique that can reverse these effects. It calms the basal ganglia, which is the area of the brain that controls anxiety. Taking deep breaths also relaxes your muscles, which relieves tension, and helps your brain function more efficiently, which improves your thinking and judgment.

Here's how you do it. As you inhale, let your belly expand. When you exhale, pull your belly in to push the air out of your lungs. This allows you to expel more air, which in turn, encourages you to inhale more deeply. Keep breathing in this fashion, and stressful feelings may diminish.

Deep-Breathing Exercise

Practice this simple three-step exercise to learn diaphragmatic breathing.

1. Lie on your back and place a small book on your belly.
2. When you inhale, make the book go up.
3. When you exhale, make the book go down.

Stress-Relieving Breathing Strategy

Whenever you feel stressed out, use this diaphragmatic breathing technique.

- Take a deep breath.
- Hold it for four to five seconds.
- Slowly blow it out (take about six to eight seconds to exhale completely).
- Take another deep breath (as deep as you can).
- Hold it for four to five seconds.
- Blow it out slowly again.
- Do this ten times (odds are you will feel relaxed).

Meditate or pray on a regular basis. Decades of research have shown that meditation and prayer calm stress, enhance brain function, and increase your self-control. Meditation has long been promoted as a way to simultaneously relax, re-energize, and develop focus. One study on the effects of meditation on addiction and relapse involved a comparison between incarcerated substance abusers who followed a traditional treatment program and those who took a course in a form of meditation. After being released from jail, the prisoners who learned to meditate showed significant reductions in alcohol, marijuana, and crack cocaine use compared to those in the traditional treatment programs.

At the Amen Clinics, we performed a SPECT study on a Kundalini Yoga form of meditation called Kirtan Kriya in which we scanned eleven people on one day when they didn't meditate and then the next day during a meditation session. The brain imaging scans taken after the meditation showed marked decreases in activity in the left parietal lobes, which showed a decreasing awareness of time and space. They also showed significant increases in activity in the prefrontal cortex, which showed that meditation helps people tune in, not out. We also observed increased activity in the right temporal lobe, an area that has been associated with spirituality.

Another brain imaging study of transcendental meditation (TM) showed calming in the anterior cingulate and basal ganglia, diminishing anxiety and worries, and fostering relaxation. Other studies have shown that it also improves attention and planning, reduces depression and anxiety, decreases sleepiness, and protects the brain from cognitive decline associated with normal aging. These findings point to real benefits for all types of addicts. Here are some of the ways meditation can help each type.

- *Type 1 Compulsive Addicts.* Meditation lowers activity in the anterior cingulate activity, which can reduce compulsivity.

- *Type 2 Impulsive Addicts.* Meditation increases activity in the prefrontal cortex and improves attention and planning, which can lower impulsivity.

- *Type 3 Impulsive-Compulsive Addicts.* See benefits for Types 1 and 2 above.

- *Type 4 Sad or Emotional Addicts.* Meditation has been found to reduce depression, which can reduce your desire to self-medicate.

- *Type 5 Anxious Addicts.* Meditation calms the basal ganglia, which can reduce your anxiety.

- *Type 6 Temporal Lobe Addicts.* Meditation has been found to activate the right temporal lobe, which may help deepen a person's sense of spirituality.

You don't need to devote big chunks of time to the practice of meditation for stress relief. In my clinical practice, I often recommend meditation as an integral part of a treatment plan. Many of my patients have reported back that they feel calmer and less stressed after just a few minutes of daily meditation. Here is a simple meditation technique that I teach my patients.

Getting Ready to Meditate

- Find a quiet place that's free of distractions. Lock the door to avoid interruptions and turn off your cell phone.

- Give yourself twelve minutes to meditate, once or twice a day, preferably before breakfast and dinner, and don't stop until this time is up. Check a clock occasionally, but don't use an alarm, as it might shock you out of your relaxation.

- Sit comfortably and consciously relax all your muscles from the bottom of your feet to the top of your head, and close your eyes. Enjoy your calm attitude as you breathe slowly and deeply from your belly.

- Try to forget all the thoughts that swirl through your mind. Put a stop to your internal monologue. Cease thinking in words. When memories arise, tell them to go away.

Daily Twelve-Minute Kirtan Kriya Meditation Practice

This twelve-minute meditation involves chanting the following simple sounds—"sa" "ta" "na" "ma"—while doing repetitive finger movements.

- Touch the thumb of each hand to the index finger while chanting "sa."

- Touch the thumb of each hand to the middle finger while chanting "ta."

- Touch the thumb of each hand to the ring finger while chanting "na."

- Touch the thumb of each hand to the pinkie finger while chanting "ma."

- Repeat the sounds for two minutes aloud.

- Repeat the sounds for two minutes whispering.

- Repeat the sounds for four minutes silently.

- Repeat the sounds for two minutes whispering.

- Repeat the sounds for two minutes aloud.

- When you finish, sit quietly for a minute or two, and try to merge your calmed mind and body with your regular mode of being. Congratulations! Now you know how to meditate.

Kirtan Kriya Fingertip Movements

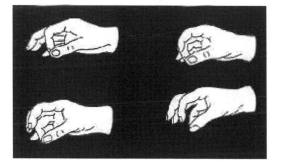

I realize that many people going through withdrawal or trying to break free from addictions may have trouble sitting quietly for twelve minutes. If this is the case, you may want to try something called the Relaxation Response developed by Herbert Benson, MD, at Harvard Medical School. This is a very simple introduction to meditation. I have found that many of my patients have managed to reduce their stress with just two minutes of meditation a day.

Two-Minute Relaxation Response Meditation

This two-minute meditation will help quiet your mind.

- Sit quietly.
- Close your eyes.
- Take slow deep breaths.
- Say the word "one" whenever you exhale.

- If your mind wanders, just bring your thoughts back to the word "one" as you exhale.

Prayer offers many of the same stress-relief benefits as meditation. Physicians Larry Dossey (*Healing Words*), Dale Matthews (*The Faith Factor*), and others have written books outlining the scientific evidence of the medical benefits of prayer and other meditative states. Some of these benefits include: reduced feelings of stress, improved sleep, reduced anxiety and depression, fewer headaches, more relaxed muscles, and longer life spans.

A 1998 Duke University study of 577 men and women hospitalized for physical illness showed that the more patients used positive spiritual coping strategies (seeking spiritual support from friends and religious leaders, having faith in God, praying), the lower their level of depressive symptoms and the higher their quality of life.

Hypnosis. When I was a medical student, I saw one of my professors hypnotize a patient. Captivated by the healing potential of hypnosis, I wanted to learn everything I could about how to use this safe and drug-free technique to help people get better. And so I took a month-long elective in how to hypnotize patients and teach them self-hypnosis. This experience turned out to be one of those pivotal events in my life that powerfully influenced the nature of my thinking and medical practice.

When I was an intern at the Walter Reed Army Medical Center in Washington, DC, I started using hypnosis to help my patients with a variety of problems. For example, some of my patients suffered from insomnia and wanted sleeping pills. But I struck a deal with all of them. I said, "Look, first I'm going to try putting you into a hypnotic trance that will help you fall asleep. I'll record a tape for you so that you can use it instead of pills. And if that doesn't work, *then* I'll give you a sleeping pill." And of all the interns that year, I prescribed half the number of sleeping pills for patients.

I had so much success with hypnosis during my internship that I have continued using it in my practice with patients ever since. I have found it to be helpful in decreasing stress, anxiety, insomnia, pain, and negative thinking patterns, all conditions that increase the potential for relapse. I have seen it work for people with addictions of all kinds, including overeating, smoking, and substance abuse. To use it effectively to battle addictions, it needs to be used in combination with a responsible treatment program or support group. For overeaters who want to lose weight, it works best when it is combined with a healthy weight-loss program.

Significant scientific evidence suggests that hypnosis can be a powerful aid to weight loss. In one scientific review comparing a series of weight-loss studies with and without hypnosis, it was found that adding hypnosis significantly improved weight loss. The average post-treatment weight loss was 6.0 pounds without hypnosis and 11.83 pounds with hypnosis, nearly double. In a further follow-up period, the mean weight loss was 6.03 pounds without hypnosis and 14.88 pounds with hypnosis. The benefits of hypnosis increased over time.

Hypnosis can help people learn positive eating behaviors and create healthy long-term patterns of food intake. Some common hypnotic suggestions I give to patients include "feel full faster... eat more slowly... savor and enjoy each bite of your food... visualize yourself at your ideal weight and body... see the behaviors you need to do to get the body you want."

Guided imagery and self-hypnosis are simple methods that I have used very successfully for decades with my patients. Now I'm going to show you how to do these.

Self-Hypnosis for Stress Relief

Use this self-hypnosis exercise when you feel stressed.

- First, find a spot on the wall a little bit above your eye level and focus on it. (If you're lying down, find a spot on the ceiling so your eyes are looking up.) What this does is take all the distractions in your head and get rid of them by focusing on a spot. So with this spot on the wall, you now have an external focus.

- Slowly count to twenty.

- Let your eyes close. As your eyes close, take three very deep, very slow breaths with your belly. As you do that, say to yourself with each inhalation, "I breathe in relaxation and warmth." With each exhale, say, "I blow out all the tension, all the worries, all the things that interfere with me becoming relaxed."

- After that third breath, keep breathing slowly and deeply, and with your eyes closed, roll them up as far as they'll go. What you're doing right now is tensing the muscles.

- After you roll them up as far as they'll go, let them come back down, and you'll notice that those muscles you tensed are now becoming relaxed. Just imagine the relaxation spreading from the top of your head all the way down to the bottom of your feet in a very slow progressive fashion.

- Now imagine yourself walking down a staircase or walking down a road, or going down an escalator. Something is moving you downwards, making your body feel even more relaxed. As you walk down a staircase or descend on the escalator, count backwards from ten.

- When you reach the number one, find yourself in your favorite place—a special place where you can go to any time you need it in your imagination. For me, it would be the beach. For you, it might be the green forest or the snowy mountains. What is your special place that has relaxation written all over it? If you could go any place in the world, where would you go?
  Write the name of it here:_____

- Now I want you to go to that place and experience it in your mind with all five of your senses to see what's there, feel what's there, to hear what's there, and to smell and taste what's there.

This is an effective, feel-good technique to reset your nervous system so that you feel ever so much more relaxed. It is very powerful. You can do this whenever you feel stressed. For example, you can close your office door and take an inner journey on your lunch break. You can do this to mellow out after a hard day or after your children have gone to bed. I have even practiced guided imagery and self-hypnosis while sitting on trains, buses, and airplanes.

On our website (www.amenclinics.com), you can find a series of hypnosis CDs and downloads that I have created for you that will guide you through this process.

Exercise to Reduce Stress

In previous chapters, you learned how exercise can improve brain function, increase self-control, and reduce cravings. Physical activity is also an effective stress reducer because it counteracts the stress response. Exercise allows your body to use up and flush out some of those chemicals that flood your system when you feel stressed. This helps decrease the negative effects of stress and allows you to get back to a relaxed state more quickly. Other types of exercise, such as yoga and t'ai chi, can counteract stress by increasing relaxation, focusing on breathing, and providing a sense of balance.

When you feel stressed, get up and take a brisk walk to get your blood moving and your heart pumping or do a few relaxing yoga poses.

Get Enough Sleep

In Chapter 9: Boost Your Brain to Get Control, you saw that lack of sleep increases the likelihood of using drugs, drinking more alcohol and caffeine, smoking more, and getting less exercise. To prevent relapse, you have to get adequate sleep, but you must be careful with the strategies you use. For people with addictions, prescription sleeping aids are NOT the answer. They can ignite the addiction circuits in the brain and either create new addictions or cause relapse. Instead, you need to focus on natural remedies that are not habit-forming.

Here are tips to help you go to sleep and stay asleep.

- Maintain a regular sleep schedule—even on weekends.

- Create a soothing nighttime routine (a warm bath, meditation, or massage).

- Don't take daytime naps.

- Listen to soothing music.

- Engage in regular exercise—just not within four hours of bedtime.

- Try self-hypnosis.

- Turn off computers and cell phones two hours before bedtime.

- Don't eat two to three hours before bedtime.

- Avoid drinking caffeinated beverages in the late afternoon or evening.

- Consider taking nonaddictive natural supplements, such as my Restful Sleep formula that contains melatonin, valerian, magnesium, B6, and GABA.

Practice Gratitude

If you want your brain to work better, be grateful for the good things in your life. Focusing on the positive things in your life can make you happier regardless of your circumstances. At the Amen Clinics, we performed a SPECT study, which found that practicing gratitude causes real changes in your brain that enhance brain function and make you feel better.

Stress-Relieving Gratitude Exercise #1

Write down five things you are grateful for every day. Use the form provided, make copies of it, or just use a notepad to write down the things you are grateful for. Writing helps to solidify them in your brain. In my experience, when depressed patients did this exercise every day, they actually needed less antidepressant medication.

5 Things I'm Grateful For Today

1. _____
2. _____
3. _____
4. _____
5. _____

Stress-Relieving Gratitude Exercise #2: The Glad Game

No matter what situation you are in, try to find something to be glad about. Think of a time when you were in a difficult or disappointing situation and started to think negatively but then found (or now can see) a "silver lining." Now, try to explain the same situation from a "glad" standpoint. What did you find to be glad about the situation?

_____

_____

_____

_____

_____

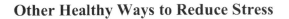

Other Healthy Ways to Reduce Stress

There are many other healthy ways to lower your stress levels. Here's a list that you can refer to when you feel overwhelmed.

- Pet your dog or cat.

- Take a warm bath.

- Learn to delegate. You don't have to do everything yourself, and it is okay to ask for help.

- Don't automatically say "yes" to every invitation, project, or activity. Say "no" to things that don't fit into your goals and desires.

- Listen to soothing music.

- Lavender has been shown to have calming, stress-relieving properties, so use lavender-scented oils, candles, sprays, lotion, or sachets.

- If you're stressed about an upcoming event or situation where you have to give a talk or meet new people, rehearse what you are going to say.

- Learn to laugh at yourself.

UNCHAIN YOUR BRAIN CHECKLIST

✓ Practice all of the stress-relieving suggestions in this chapter to find which ones work best for you.

✓ If you find yourself in a stressful situation, use deep breathing to calm down.

✓ Start your day with a brief meditation to set a peaceful and calm tone for the day.

✓ Try self-hypnosis to help you relax or fall asleep.

✓ Make exercise a regular habit to improve your body's ability to handle the stress response.

✓ Focus on natural remedies to get more restful sleep.

✓ Be grateful for the positive things in your life and always look for the bright side of any situation.

✓ When stress is overwhelming, consider non-addictive natural supplements to promote calm.

✓ Keep a list of healthy stress-relievers nearby for times when you feel like you might lose control.

Chapter 14

Step #9

H-A-L-T PLUS

Overcome the Barriers That Keep You From Conquering Your Addictions

Don't let other people, places, or things take control of your behavior.

I recently became a grandfather for the first time and couldn't wait to visit my new grandchild. When I went to my daughter's home, one of my friends was visiting her too. She asked me if I wanted something to eat, and I said no, I wasn't hungry. I thought that would be the end of that discussion, but she continued to ask me an additional five times if I wanted something to eat!

Sandra, thirty-one, is one of my patients who has started doing a highly aerobic salsa dance class three times a week in the evenings in an effort to boost her brain, reduce cravings for cocaine, and prevent relapse. But on the nights when her class meets, her boyfriend Jeremy tries to coax her to stay home and watch a movie with him instead.

Brooke, twenty-two, wants to optimize her brain so she can stop her sad and emotional overeating, and she knows that taking a multivitamin, fish oil, and vitamin D could help. But she's worried about the cost of high-quality supplements so she doesn't get the mood-boosting nutrients she needs and continues to overeat.

When you are healing from addiction, you will face a number of daily obstacles that jeopardize your brain health and recovery. Pushers, energy zappers, money concerns—these are some of the things that can stand in the way of your efforts to improve your brain health and prevent relapse.

When you start living a brain healthy life free of addictions, it can make those around you uncomfortable, especially if they have addictions or a lot of bad brain habits of their own. Deep down, some people—even those who love you the most—don't want you to succeed because it will make them feel like more of a failure. For others, their habits are so ingrained that they simply don't know how to react to your new lifestyle. Many of my patients notice this kind of behavior with their families, friends, and coworkers. This is why it is so important for you to take control of your life and recovery. You need to be prepared for the obstacles that will come your way so you can deal with them.

You will be better prepared to handle challenges if you live by the acronym H-A-L-T, which is a common term used in addiction treatment programs. H-A-L-T stands for:

- Don't get too **Hungry.** Eat frequent, small, high-quality meals and take nutritional supplements to optimize your brain and balance your blood sugar. See Chapter 11: Eat Right to Think Right and Heal from Your Addiction for more on brain healthy eating.

- Don't get too **Angry.** Maintain control over your emotions and don't let negative thinking patterns rule your life. See Chapter 12: Kill the Addiction ANTs That Infest Your Brain and Keep You in Chains for more details on changing your thinking.

- Don't get too **Lonely.** Social skills and a positive social network are critical to maintaining freedom from addiction. Enlist a team of supporters and healthy role models.

- Don't get too **Tired.** Make sleep a priority to boost brain function and improve judgment and self-control.

Don't Let Pushers Sabotage Your Brain Healthy Life and Recovery

People, companies, and our society will try to push things on you that threaten your brain healthy ways and trigger your addiction. As a society, we're bombarded with messages about food, coffee, cigarettes, gambling, sex, alcohol, and more. TV commercials, billboards, and radio ads are constantly showing us images of happy, attractive people enjoying greasy fast food, judgment-impairing cocktails, and dehydrating caffeinated drinks that reduce brain function and self-control. Movies depict gorgeous celebrities smoking, drinking, and doing drugs, which can fire up those emotional memory centers in the brain and trigger relapse.

Corporate America is highly skilled at pushing people to eat and drink things that are not good for our brain health. Restaurants and fast-food joints train employees to "upsell" as a way to increase sales and subsequently, expand our waistlines. Here are some of the sneaky tactics food sellers use to try to get you to eat and drink more.

"Do you want to supersize that for only 39 cents?"

"Do you want fries with your meal?"

"Do you want bread first?"
(This makes you hungrier so you eat more!)

"Do you want an appetizer?"

"Do you want another drink?"

"Do you want a larger drink? It is a better deal!"

Your response to all of these questions should always be, "No!" Eating or drinking more than you need just because it's more economical will cost you far more in the long run.

Unfortunately, spouses, friends, coworkers, neighbors, and even children can also make it very difficult for you to stay on track regardless of what you are addicted to. A friend who smokes may light up in front of you even though you are trying to quit. A neighbor might show up with a box of home-baked brownies for your birthday when you are trying to curb your sugar intake. At work, the receptionist may hand out candy every time you walk by, your supervisor may invite your team to go to happy hour for drinks, or a guy in the operations department may come around with a March Madness pool asking if you want to place a bet.

And of course, there are the real drug pushers—the people on school campuses, in bars and clubs, at work, or on the streets selling pot, cocaine, Ecstasy, meth, and off-label Adderall. Then there are the inadvertent pushers—the parents who keep unused prescription painkillers in unlocked medicine cabinets, store household chemicals under the kitchen sink, and leave alcohol readily available in the family room wet bar.

People aren't the only pushers. Places and environmental cues can trigger addictive behaviors. Almost everywhere you go, you will see reminders of your addiction and things that tempt you to engage in behaviors that are not brain healthy. In the addiction field, they are called "slippery places." Go to the movies and you'll have to drive by the fast food place where you used to hang out with your friends and get high. Take a cruise to Alaska because you want to see the beautiful scenery, and you'll have to face unbelievably copious amounts of food and desserts at the buffet and free-flowing alcohol. Join your colleagues at a convention in Las Vegas and you'll have to deal with all sorts of temptations that threaten your brain health and recovery. See Chapter 10: Craving Control for more information on how to deal with the urges that arise from environmental cues.

Learning to deal with and say "no" to all of these pushers in the home, on the town, at work, and at school is critical to your success.

15 Tips For Dealing With Pushers

1. Ask your family to lock up anything that might tempt you.

2. If you are going to a dinner with friends or family, call ahead to inform the host that you are on a special diet and won't be able to eat certain foods or drink alcohol.

3. If Sam in accounting was your cocaine supplier, don't walk past his office… EVER.

4. When invited to parties where people may be smoking, drinking, or doing drugs, either don't go or go with a friend who supports you in your efforts and will take you home if you feel tempted.

5. Be upfront with food pushers. Explain that you are trying to eat a more balanced diet, and that when they offer you cake, chips, or pizza, it makes it more difficult for you.

6. Instead of going out for a smoke break or drinks with friends, choose activities that aren't centered on your addiction, such as going for a walk.

7. If your coworkers invite you to happy hour, but you don't want them to push you to drink alcohol and you don't want to let them know you are in recovery, ask the bartender to put fizzy water or juice in a bar glass and garnish it with something that makes it look like an alcoholic drink.

8. When people offer seconds, tell them you are full. If they insist, explain that you are trying to watch your calories. If they continue to push extra helpings on you, ask them why they are bent on sabotaging your efforts to be healthy.

9. I know some people who will accept a piece of cake or a cocktail and then toss it in the trash or the sink as soon as the host turns away. It is better to be wasteful on occasion than to endanger your recovery.

10. Avoid visiting coworkers who have candy on their desk, and if possible, choose a route that doesn't go past the break room or the vending machines.

11. Tell your host you don't drink alcohol... period.

12. With hosts you don't know well and likely won't see again, consider telling them you have a medical problem, such as a food allergy so they won't insist you try their food.

13. Take a healthy sack lunch so you don't have to eat from the cafeteria at work or school.

14. Commit to taking control of your own body and don't let other people make you fat and stupid.

15. Be honest with pushers. Tell them you are in recovery and ask them not to offer you things that could trigger relapse.

The Three Circles: Know When You're Safe, When You're Vulnerable, and When You're in Danger

It is absolutely critical that you know what helps keep you on track with your recovery, what makes you more likely to relapse, and what puts you in imminent danger of relapse. To help my patients understand the people, places, and things that are helping their recovery and those that are putting them at greater risk for relapse, I use an exercise called the Three Circles.

For this exercise, I have my patients take a page, draw three circles on it, and label them "Red Circle," "Yellow Circle," and "Green Circle." In the green circle, I have them write down all the things that help them stay on track with their recovery. In the yellow circle, they put things that make them more vulnerable to getting off track. In the red circle, they list their danger zones—the things that put them in imminent danger of relapse.

Following is an example of what the Three Circles might look like for someone who is addicted to online pornography. Then there is a blank form called "My Three Circles" that you can use to identify what helps keep you safe, what makes you more vulnerable, and what puts you in danger. Keep this page with you to help remind you what's helping your recovery and what is putting it at risk.

THE THREE CIRCLES

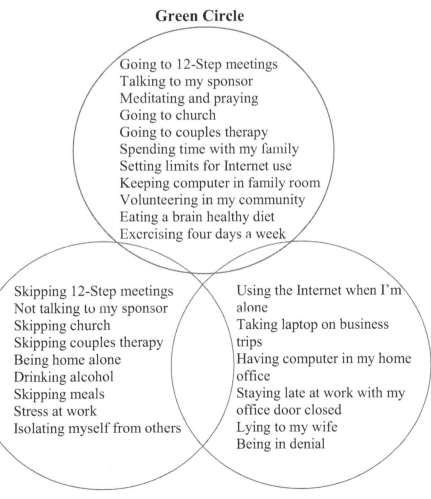

Green Circle

Going to 12-Step meetings
Talking to my sponsor
Meditating and praying
Going to church
Going to couples therapy
Spending time with my family
Setting limits for Internet use
Keeping computer in family room
Volunteering in my community
Eating a brain healthy diet
Exercising four days a week

Skipping 12-Step meetings
Not talking to my sponsor
Skipping church
Skipping couples therapy
Being home alone
Drinking alcohol
Skipping meals
Stress at work
Isolating myself from others

Using the Internet when I'm alone
Taking laptop on business trips
Having computer in my home office
Staying late at work with my office door closed
Lying to my wife
Being in denial

Yellow Circle   **Red Circle**

243

MY THREE CIRCLES

Green Circle
*In this circle, write what helps keep
you safe and on track with your recovery.*

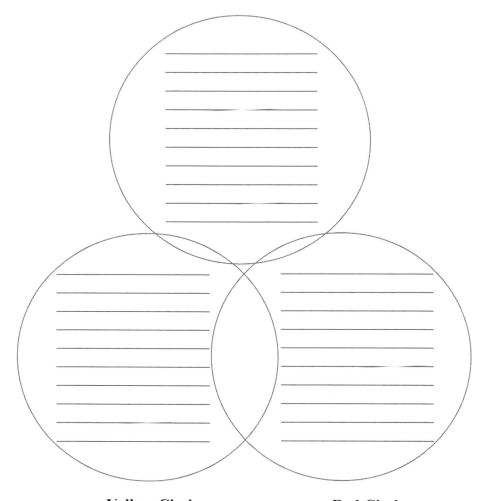

Yellow Circle
*In this circle, write what makes
you more vulnerable to relapse.*

Red Circle
*In this circle, write what puts
you in danger of relapse.*

Don't Let Energy Zappers Prevent You From Getting the Exercise You Need

The people around you may get in the way of your commitment to exercise. Your significant other may try to get you to stay in bed and cuddle in the morning instead of getting up to do your workout. You might be on your way to the gym when your kids say they want a ride somewhere NOW. Your boss might put a last-minute project on your desk just as you were about to leave work to go play basketball. Don't give in to these people. Schedule another time to get romantic with your partner. Tell your kids you will give them a ride after you have worked out. And let your boss know you had a prior commitment, but you will work on the new project later that night.

When an energy zapper tries to keep you from exercising, let them know why it's important to you and why it is also beneficial to them. Arm yourself with responses like these:

"I'm exercising because it makes me feel good and helps keep me healthy by preventing cravings and relapse. If you care about me and my health, you won't ask me to skip it."

"Physical activity puts me in a better mood, which will help our relationship and make me a better partner/friend."

"If I go exercise for an hour, I will think much more clearly afterward and will do a better job on this project."

The people around you aren't the only energy zappers. There are many other things that will rob you of energy, including:

- Inherited brain disorders
- Infectious causes
- Hormonal issues
- Anemia
- Brain trauma
- Environmental toxins

- Many medications
- Chronic stress
- Untreated past emotional trauma
- Caffeine
- Smoking
- Poor eating habits
- Poor sleep
- Too much alcohol
- Lack of exercise
- Low/erratic blood sugar states from any cause

Things that will boost your energy include:

- Treat the energy robbers described above.
- Get at least seven hours of sleep.
- Eat a brain healthy diet.
- Maintain a level blood sugar.
- Exercise four to five times a week.
- Use stress-reduction techniques.
- Test and optimize hormone levels.
- Meditate.
- Eat low-calorie, high-fiber foods (fruits, vegetables, beans, and whole grains).
- Drink green tea, which includes theanine.
- Take natural supplements, such as ashwagandha and green tea leaf extract.

Don't Let Money Concerns Stand in the Way of Brain Health

Addiction is expensive. It can wipe out your savings and ruin your credit. Money woes are very common among people with addictions. Fortunately, I can tell you that living a brain healthy life doesn't have to cost a lot of money. In fact, many of the tips in this book are absolutely free. Just check the following list for inexpensive ways to boost your brain.

50 Free and Low-Cost Ways to Improve Brain Health

1. Loving your brain is free.

2. Talking about the brain with family, friends, coworkers, and classmates is free.

3. Learning something from articles and TV features about the brain is free.

4. Keeping a daily journal to track your brain healthy habits is free.

5. Becoming aware of the various brain systems is free.

6. Understanding your own brain and how it affects your life is free.

7. Avoiding activities at high risk for brain injury is free.

8. Not buying drugs saves you money.

9. Limiting your exposure to toxins like nail polish and hair chemicals is free.

10. Cooking healthy food at home can be less expensive than eating out.

11. Buying frozen fruits in bulk is an inexpensive way to get your antioxidants.

12. Buying frozen vegetables in bulk is a low-cost option.

13. Stocking up on brain healthy beans is an inexpensive way to get more fiber in your diet.

14. Skipping the candy, cookies, and ice cream lowers your food bill.

15. Eating fewer calories costs less.

16. Eating five or six small meals doesn't cost any more than eating three big meals.

17. Saying "no" to supersizing your meal saves money.

18. At restaurants, splitting meals cuts the check in half.

19. Skipping the appetizers and desserts lowers your check.

20. Cutting out the alcohol can significantly reduce your dinner tab or bar tab.

21. Quitting smoking saves money spent on cigarettes.

22. Getting more sleep is free.

23. Drinking water costs less than drinking energy drinks, coffee, or sodas.

24. Exercising outdoors is free.

25. Thinking positive thoughts is free.

26. Cutting TV time is free.

27. Limiting video game playing is free.

28. Buying fewer video games saves money.

29. Eliminating Internet pornography sites saves money.

30. Limiting texting can save money.

31. Cutting caffeine can trim your Starbucks bill.

32. Getting books from the library for new learning is free.

33. Getting foreign language CDs from the library is free.

34. Games and puzzles are low-cost mental workouts.

35. Classes at local community colleges and the Learning Annex are relatively inexpensive.

36. Improving at your favorite activities can be free.

37. Shaking up your daily routine is free.

38. Surrounding yourself with smart people is free.

39. Meditation is free.

40. Prayer is free.

41. Saying "no" to invitations that don't serve your goals is free.

42. Being grateful is free.

43. Deep breathing for stress reduction is free.

44. Self-hypnosis is free.

45. Soothing music doesn't require a big investment.

46. Focusing on positive memories is free.

47. Talking back to your ANTs is free.

48. Writing down your goals is free.

49. Staying focused on what motivates you is free.

50. Saying "no" to pushers who want you to do unhealthy things is free.

On the other hand, there are times when it is well worth it to spend money on your brain health and recovery. Don't skimp when it comes to the following:

- Choosing a treatment program for addiction.

- Getting a complete physical to check for medical conditions that might be affecting your brain health and your addiction.

- Taking the necessary supplements to optimize your brain, control cravings, and reduce the risk for relapse.

- Seeing a professional to diagnose and treat possible brain disorders.

When seeking professional help for addiction, remember that it is important to find the right program for your needs rather than seeking out the one that charges the least amount of money. The right facility or program can have a very positive impact on your recovery and your life. The wrong program can leave you in chains. Saving money upfront can cost you in the long run. The right help is not only cost effective but also saves you unnecessary pain and suffering.

Change is Hard Work—How to Stay on Track

Change is an uncomfortable process. In fact, changing your behavior can be one of the toughest things you will ever do. The steps in this book are designed to help in your efforts to change, but don't expect it to be easy. Here are a few tips that can help you stay on the right path.

Don't try to change everything at once. If you have come to the decision that you want to make changes in your life, you probably want them to happen NOW! But after nearly thirty years of helping patients navigate the change process, I have learned that taking a gradual approach is the surest way to success. So many people try to change all at once, but this almost inevitably invites disappointment and failure. You can't change dozens of behaviors at once. Start with a few vital behaviors—the ones that will have the biggest immediate impact—and go from there.

Set SMART goals. Setting the right kind of goals can help you achieve those goals and reduce the risk of failure. SMART goals are:

- **S**pecific
- **M**easurable
- **A**ttainable
- **R**ealistic
- **T**imely

Specific: You have a better chance of achieving a specific goal rather than a vague goal. For example, *"Eat oatmeal with blueberries for breakfast instead of fast food"* is a better goal than *"Eat better."*

Measurable: When you can measure your goals, it is easier to know if you are on the right path to achieving them and lets you know when you have reached your goal. For example, *"Go to the gym four times a week for thirty minutes each session"* is a better goal than *"Get in shape."*

Attainable: Set short-term goals that you are capable of achieving. These short-term goals will help keep you motivated toward your long-term goals. Setting goals that are too lofty or long term can be demotivating. For example, *"Lose one hundred pounds in one year"* sounds impossible. *"Lose two pounds a week"* doesn't sound so hard, but it will get you to that bigger goal. When you give yourself attainable short-term goals, it makes it easier for you to believe in your ability to change. In order to change, you must believe in your ability to make it happen. If you don't believe, you'll never do it.

Realistic: Goals that are unrealistic set you up to feel like a failure. For example, *"Be a rock star"* may be completely

251

unrealistic if you don't play a musical instrument, can't sing, don't write songs, aren't in a band, and aren't willing to devote hours and hours to rehearsing. A realistic goal is one that you are both willing and able to work hard to achieve. If you love music, your goal might be *"Get a job in the music industry by interning at a record label during college and learning everything I can about the business."*

Timely: Goals without a timeframe lack urgency. Set a specific timeframe, such as *"by March 15,"* to force you into action.

Believe you can do it. If you don't believe in yourself, you will never achieve your goals. Take what you learned from Chapter 12: Kill the Addiction ANTs That Infest Your Brain and Keep You in Chains and start changing your negative thinking patterns to honest and positive thinking to help you believe in yourself.

Reward yourself for the small successes. When you reach short-term goals, give yourself a pat on the back, but don't celebrate with substances or activities that harm your brain. Find brain healthy ways to reward yourself, such as buying yourself a new book, taking a warm bath, or getting a massage.

Don't trade one addiction for another. Did you know that the leading cause of death among recovering alcoholics is tobacco-related illness? The rate of smoking among recovering alcoholics is more than triple that of the general population. People in Alcoholics Anonymous also consume more coffee than the general public. Why do so many people who are trying to break free from their addictions simply quit one bad habit and acquire another one in its place?

In many cases, there are underlying bio-psycho-social-spiritual reasons for the addiction. And when you remove the addictive substance or behavior, but do NOT address all four pillars of addiction, you can't heal. You will look for other ways to self-medicate. To be truly free from addiction, you need to treat all four pillars of addiction and stay away from all addictive substances.

Get back on track—setbacks don't mean failure. The road to change is not a one-way street. The steps to change are not static. I frequently tell my patients that their journey will be like going up and down a staircase. They will go up several steps, feel like they've made progress, then go back down a few steps when difficult situations arise. They will make several more steps of progress, then slip back a few, but usually not as many as before. Usually, the slope of progress is in an upward, positive direction.

If you aren't expecting to encounter setbacks, it can derail your efforts. Let's say you're trying to get a handle on your caffeine consumption. You've been doing great, cutting back to only one cup of coffee in the morning. But after pulling an all-nighter before a big deadline, you find yourself nodding off at your desk in the afternoon so you head to the nearest Starbucks for a venti latte. Then you feel like you've blown it, so you get another coffee after dinner and then give up entirely on changing. Understanding that setbacks are part of the process and planning how to deal with them makes them easier to handle. So you had that extra coffee in the afternoon—just get back onto your program the next day.

Remember that change never stops. The world and people around us change constantly. With every change that comes into your life, you have the power to be in control of your behavior or to let your behavior control you.

Dealing With Obstacles

To prepare yourself for the barriers to brain health and recovery, use the chart below to write down your obstacles and plans to deal with them.

My Obstacles to Brain Health and Recovery	How I Will Deal With These Obstacles
_____	_____
_____	_____

_____   _____

_____   _____

_____   _____

UNCHAIN YOUR BRAIN CHECKLIST

- ✓ Live by the acronym H-A-L-T Plus.

- ✓ Don't let other people control your behavior.

- ✓ Don't skimp on your recovery—your life is on the line.

- ✓ Don't expect change to be easy.

- ✓ Set SMART goals to improve your chances of success.

- ✓ Celebrate your successes in brain healthy ways.

- ✓ Prepare for setbacks.

- ✓ Don't trade one addiction for another.

- ✓ Remember that change never stops.

- ✓ Plan how you will deal with obstacles.

Chapter 15

Step #10

GET WELL,
BEYOND YOURSELF

Finding Meaning in Family and Community
Addiction is a family disease.

James, eighteen, seemed to have it all—he came from a very wealthy family with an ocean-front home, was extremely bright, and had gotten accepted to a highly selective small liberal arts college on the East Coast. In his senior year in high school, he often got bored in class because it wasn't challenging enough for him. He wanted to "expand his mind" and started experimenting with drugs. By the time he went off to college, he had already gotten hooked on cocaine and meth. At college, he quickly figured out who the other drug addicts were and made friends with them. He came to think of them as his "true family" because they were the only ones who understood him.

When James would go home to visit his parents and two older sisters, he barely spoke to them because they no longer had anything in common. All James was interested in was getting high; he didn't care about the family activities he used to enjoy, like sailing or hiking. When the money his parents sent each month no longer covered his drug habit, he started selling drugs to make money. One day, he sold cocaine to an undercover cop on campus and got arrested.

After his arrest, James made a harsh discovery. His "true family" of drug addict friends never came to visit him, made no effort to contact him, and offered no support throughout his ordeal. In fact, James found out that when they learned he was in jail, they went to his dorm room and stole his things to help pay for their drugs.

On the other hand, his family back home moved across the country to stay in a hotel so they could be near James and hired a hot-shot lawyer to handle his case. James ended up getting sentenced to six months in jail and mandatory drug treatment. The only people who visited him in jail were his parents and his two sisters. His parents researched addiction treatment programs and sent James to one near their home so they could take part in weekly family therapy sessions.

It didn't take long for James to realize that the friends he thought were his "true family" really didn't care about him at all. They only cared about drugs. His real family loved him and helped him through the healing process so he could kick his drug habit and get back to the life he used to enjoy.

Chantal, sixteen, was hooked on booze, OxyContin, and the sleeping pill Ambien. She would drink and pop OxyContin all day long and would take five Ambien in the morning, five more in the afternoon, and another five in the evening. When her parents found her stash, they dropped her off at a treatment program and told the staff to "fix her." Chantal's nineteen-year-old sister had already gone through treatment for addiction to painkillers and was currently going to college abroad. Her older sister was still taking painkillers and her parents knew it, but they continued to send her money and pay her bills anyway.

On family day at the treatment center, Chantal sat by herself because her parents were too busy to come. Chantal didn't really care because she didn't want them there anyway. Her parents actually had problems of their own with drugs and alcohol but were in complete denial. Her father drank too much, and her mother used prescription painkillers and sleeping pills on a regular basis. That's where Chantal first got the pills—from her mother's medicine cabinet. Her dad had started giving her wine and cocktails with dinner at home when she was about twelve and would let her drink any time they had a party at the house.

When Chantal left treatment and went back home, she found more pills in her mother's medicine cabinet and lots of alcohol in the kitchen. It wasn't long before she went back to drinking and popping pills, but this time, tragically, she overdosed and died at the age of seventeen.

James and Chantal are examples of how your family impacts your recovery. In Chantal's case, she was never able to heal in part because she didn't want her parents to get involved in her recovery and because her parents were in denial about their own problems and how they were contributing to Chantal's troubles. With James, his family got involved in his treatment and did everything they could to guide him onto a new path. And James allowed them to be a part of his recovery.

Getting your family involved with your treatment and recovery is an essential part of the healing process whether you are a parent, stepparent, sibling, or child. It is important to include your family in therapy so they can understand how to help you live a life free of addiction.

Addiction Runs in Families and Ruins Families

As you learned earlier, your family genetics play a role in your risk for addiction. If one or more people in your family have a problem with addiction, it's more likely that you will too. And if you have an addiction, it's quite possible that someone else in your family may have problems with addictive behavior as well.

In my practice, I often meet with families who are dealing with multiple family members who have substance abuse problems. It can be one or both of the parents, one or more of the children, and even grandparents, aunts, uncles, or siblings. When I meet with a patient who is suffering from addiction, I always ask about their family history and whether or not anyone else in the family has had problems with addiction. In many cases, the answer is yes.

Just as your family can influence your addiction, your addiction can impact your family. Family members typically complain that the substance abusers in the family are erratic, selfish, and unpredictable. That puts everyone else in the family on edge and creates an environment of chronic stress. I have also found that parents who drink regularly tend to be less available for their children and less able to see to their needs.

For parents, having an adolescent child with an addiction can absolutely ruin your family life. As a parent, it makes you feel like garbage. Other parents are saying, "My kid's going to Princeton," and you're thinking, "My kid's going to rehab." What they're really saying is, "I'm a good parent, and you're a bad parent." Nobody would say, "Your kid has diabetes, so you're a bad parent." But our society is cruel about addiction.

Parents of addicts go through deep despair wondering, "What did I do wrong?" Or they blame their spouse saying, "It's your fault because your Dad was an alcoholic." Having a child who is addicted is the biggest challenge a parent will ever face. You can't walk away from your child. You can walk away from a husband, wife, boyfriend, girlfriend, friend, or coworker, but you can never walk away from your child.

Treating Addiction is a Family Affair

To improve your chances of preventing relapse, you have to get your whole family involved in your treatment. Many people, like Chantal's parents, mistakenly believe that they can just drop off their child, spouse, or sibling at a treatment facility and say, "Fix him" or "Fix her." But that doesn't work. These folks are often very afraid of the consequences of getting involved.

They may be terrified that someone will point out that they have played a role in the problem, or that they have an addiction problem themselves. Sometimes they are terrified that if their own problems are brought to the surface, their status in the community could be negatively affected. Other people may feel so much shame, guilt, and humiliation that they are too embarrassed to take part in the process. What I always say is family members have to become part of the solution and stop being part of the problem.

To heal one person, the whole family must be healed. Family members have to examine their own behaviors to determine how they might be contributing to the problem and be willing to change their ways. They need to get involved in the addicted person's treatment and recovery by attending family day events at treatment centers, participating in family therapy or couples therapy, and accompanying them to support groups. And they have to stop being an inadvertent "pusher" or enabler.

Scientific research has found that people with substance abuse problems who engage in couples therapy or family therapy rather than just individual therapy are less likely to relapse. This shows that family bonding can be a very powerful ally in your efforts to stay away from the substances and behaviors that hurt you. It provides the foundation for the social support that is one of the four pillars of healing.

If you want to prevent relapse, you also need to widen your social support network and create an "extended family" of people who are living a brain healthy lifestyle. Interacting with other people in recovery who are committed to good health will encourage you to stick with the new habits you have adopted. When you surround yourself with like-minded people, it makes a positive difference in your health and well-being. Join support groups to find other people you can lean on and learn from.

Create a Brain Healthy Family

Creating a brain healthy family is critical for successful recovery, whether it is a parent or child who is trying to break free from addiction. To improve brain health in your household, take the advice in this book and apply it to your family. Here are some practical ways to do it.

- *Love your brain.* Teach your family members about the brain and how important it is in their day-to-day life.

- *Protect your brain.* Don't let family members take part in risky activities that increase the risk of brain injuries.

- *Feed your brain.* Serve nutritious meals that nourish the brain and body and don't keep junk food at home.

- *Rest your brain.* Keep regular sleep schedules for children and parents.

- *Work your brain.* Encourage new learning at home.

- *Exercise for your brain.* Engage in physical activities as a family.

- *De-stress your brain.* Teach children and adults how to deal with daily stress in healthy ways.

- *Kill the ANTs.* Teach family members how to talk back to negative thoughts.

- *Serenade your brain.* Have family music nights where you sing and play musical instruments.

- *Treat brain problems early.* See a professional if any family member is showing signs of mental health issues.

Here are some basic principles that parents and partners need to keep in mind.

- The brain is involved in everything your family does.

- How the members of your family think, feel, act, and interact has to do with the moment-by-moment functioning of your brains.

- When the brains in your family work right, your family tends to be effective, thoughtful, and energetic.

- When the brains in your family are troubled, your family can have problems with depression, anxiety, work or school performance, impulsivity, anger, inflexibility, memory, relationships, and addiction.

- Brain dysfunction, even when subtle, may be getting in the way of your family and individual success.

- Optimizing the brains in your family optimizes both individual and family success.

Seven Steps Parents Can Take NOW to Prevent Addiction

1. *You need a relationship to have influence.* You need to devote time to developing your relationship with your children, and you must have a willingness to listen to them.

2. *Be your children's parent, not their best friend.* Children and adolescents need supervision. You have to be your children's frontal lobes until theirs fully develops around age twenty-five.

3. *Treat underlying problems, such as trauma, anxiety, ADD, or depression.* These brain disorders are associated with a higher incidence of addiction. Treating them can lower that risk.

4. *Do not enable them but teach them self-control.* Children need to understand that there are consequences to their actions, and they need to learn to delay gratification.

5. *Educate your children.* My children are very vulnerable to addictions because there is a long line of serious alcohol abuse in their mother's family. I have told them that if they never drink they will never have a problem, but if they drink it is like Russian roulette, and they may have a very serious problem.

6. *Do not let them engage in, or model for them, "thrilling to death" behavior.* Take time to relax, spend time together, pray, and meditate together. Build up the pleasure centers in the brain; do not wear them out. Children develop their preferences and habits in life based on exposure. What you feed kids, how much you drink at dinner, how you react to stress, whether or not you smoke, the amount of TV and video games you allow them to play —these set up lifelong habits and preferences. It is critical to set up proper modeling for children and teens so they can learn healthy brain-boosting skills.

7. *Do not introduce them to drinking and drugs at home.* I have worked with a lot of patients who told me that their parents smoked pot with them at age eight or offered alcohol to them as teens. It is NOT better if you drink or do drugs with your child at home rather than letting them discover these things elsewhere. Also, be sure to keep all prescription drugs locked away where children can't access them. It is also a good idea to lock up inhalants, which include a variety of common household items, such as spray paint, aerosol sprays, glue, and cleaning fluids.

Stop Thinking About Yourself and Start Helping Others

In addition to getting your family involved in your recovery, it is important to get involved with your family and your community. People with active addictions tend to balance poor self-esteem with extreme narcissism. There are a few common sayings in the addiction field that sum up this self-absorption: *"I'm not much, but I'm all I think about"* and *"Enough about me, what do you think about me?"*

When you stop focusing on yourself and start looking outside yourself, you have reached the final stage in the recovery process. Learning to give back to your friends, family, and community through service provides the spiritual therapy that completes the four pillars of addiction and healing. Volunteering and serving others puts you back in touch with your core values and gives you

262

a sense of purpose in life. It helps you feel like your life matters, and that is one of the best ways to break free of your addictions for good.

If the notion of volunteering is new to you, here are ten simple ways you can give back.

- Do someone else's chores around the house.

- Serve meals at a local homeless shelter.

- Participate in a charity walk or run. (It helps the charity and helps you get the exercise you need.)

- Visit patients in a local hospital or senior living facility.

- Walk dogs at a local shelter.

- Volunteer to pick up litter at local parks, beaches, mountains, or wilderness areas.

- Pull up weeds and plant flowers at a local school or church.

- Read books to children for story time at a library.

- Rake leaves, shovel snow, or do household repairs for an elderly neighbor.

- Offer to play guitar or sing during church services on Sundays.

UNCHAIN YOUR BRAIN CHECKLIST

- ✓ Recognize that addiction runs in families.

- ✓ Be aware that you aren't the only one affected by your addiction.

- ✓ Get your entire family involved in your treatment and recovery.

- ✓ Commit yourself to improving the brain health of your whole family.

- ✓ Take steps NOW to prevent addiction in your children.

- ✓ Seek friendships with other people who are living a brain healthy life.

- ✓ Give back to your family, friends, neighbors, and community.

Appendix A

UNCHAIN YOUR BRAIN
MASTER QUESTIONNAIRE

Copyright © 2010 Daniel Amen, M.D.

Please rate yourself on each of the symptoms listed below using the following scale. If possible, to give yourself the most complete picture, have another person who knows you well (such as a spouse, lover, or parent) rate you as well. List other person_____

0 = Never
1 = Rarely
2 = Occasionally
3 = Frequently
4 = Very Frequently
NA = Not Applicable/known

Other Self

_____ _____ 1.   Trouble sustaining attention
_____ _____ 2.   Lacks attention to detail
_____ _____ 3.   Easily distracted
_____ _____ 4.   Procrastinate until I have to do something
_____ _____ 5.   Restless
_____ _____ 6.   Loses things
_____ _____ 7.   Difficulty expressing empathy for others
_____ _____ 8.   Blurts out answers, interrupts frequently
_____ _____ 9.   Impulsive (saying or doing things without thinking first)
_____ _____ 10. Needs caffeine or nicotine in order to focus
_____ _____ 11. Gets stuck on negative thoughts
_____ _____ 12. Worries excessively
_____ _____ 13. Tendency toward compulsive or addictive behaviors

_____ _____ 14. Holds grudges
_____ _____ 15. Upset when things do not go your way
_____ _____ 16. Upset when things are out of place
_____ _____ 17. Tendency to be oppositional or argumentative
_____ _____ 18. Dislikes change
_ __ _____ 19. Needing to have things done a certain way or you become very upset
_____ _____ 20. Trouble seeing options in situations
_____ _____ 21. Feeling sad
_____ _____ 22. Being negative
_____ _____ 23. Feeling dissatisfied
_____ _____ 24. Feeling bored
_____ _____ 25. Low energy
_____ _____ 26. Decreased interest in things that are usually fun or pleasurable
_____ _____ 27. Feelings of hopelessness, helplessness, worthlessness, or guilt
_____ _____ 28. Crying spells
_____ _____ 29. Chronic low self-esteem
_____ _____ 30. Social isolation
_____ _____ 31. Feelings of nervousness and anxiety
_____ _____ 32. Feelings of panic
_____ _____ 33. Symptoms of heightened muscle tension, such as headaches or sore muscles
_____ _____ 34. Tendency to predict the worst
_____ _____ 35. Avoid conflict
_____ _____ 36. Excessive fear of being judged or scrutinized by others
_____ _____ 37. Excessive motivation, trouble stopping work
_____ _____ 38. Lacks confidence in their abilities
_____ _____ 39. Always watching for something bad to happen
_____ _____ 40. Easily startled
_____ _____ 41. Temper problems
_____ _____ 42. Short fuse
_____ _____ 43. Irritability tends to build, then explodes, then recedes, often tired after a rage
_____ _____ 44. Unstable or unpredictable moods
_____ _____ 45. Misinterprets comments as negative when they are not

_____ _____ 46. Déjà vu (feelings of being somewhere you have never been)

_____ _____ 47. Often feel as though others are watching you or out to hurt you

_____ _____ 48. Dark or violent thoughts, that may come out of the blue

_____ _____ 49. Trouble finding the right word to say

_____ _____ 50. Headaches or abdominal pain of uncertain origin

_____ _____ 51. Tend to be clumsy or accident prone

_____ _____ 52. Walks into furniture or walls

_____ _____ 53. Trouble with coordination

_____ _____ 54. Poor handwriting

_____ _____ 55. Trouble maintaining an organized work area

_____ _____ 56. Multiple piles around the house

_____ _____ 57. More sensitive to noise than others

_____ _____ 58. Particularly sensitive to touch or tags in clothing

_____ _____ 59. Trouble learning new information or routines

_____ _____ 60. Trouble keeping up in conversations

_____ _____ 61. Forgetful

_____ _____ 62. Memory problems

_____ _____ 63. Trouble remembering appointments

_____ _____ 64. Trouble remembering to take medications or supplements

_____ _____ 65. Trouble remembering things that happened recently

_____ _____ 66. Trouble remembering names

_____ _____ 67. It is hard for me to memorize things for school, work, or hobbies

_____ _____ 68. I know something one day but do not remember it to the next

_____ _____ 69. I forget what I am going to say right in the middle of saying it

_____ _____ 70. I have trouble following directions that have more than one or two steps

_____ _____ 71. Have trouble sleeping

_____ _____ 72. Snores loudly or others complain about your snoring

_____ _____ 73. Other say you stop breathing when you sleep

_____ _____ 74. Feel fatigued or tired during the day
_____ _____ 75. Crave sweets during the day
_____ _____ 76. Agitated, easily upset, nervous when meals are missed
_____ _____ 77. Get lightheaded if meals are missed
_____ _____ 78. Eating relieves fatigue
_____ _____ 79. Light sensitive and bothered by glare, sunlight, headlights, or streetlights
_____ _____ 80. Become tired and/or experience headaches, mood changes, feel restless, or have an inability to stay focused with bright or fluorescent lights
_____ _____ 81. Have trouble reading words that are on white, glossy paper
_____ _____ 82. When reading, words or letters shift, shake, blur, move, run together, disappear, or become difficult to perceive
_____ _____ 83. Feel tense, tired, sleepy, or even get headaches with reading
_____ _____ 84. Have problems judging distance and have difficulty with such things as escalators, stairs, ball sports, or driving
_____ _____ 85. Night driving is hard
_____ _____ 86. Craving for simple carbohydrates, such as bread, pasta, cookies, or candy
_____ _____ 87. Winter depression (mood problems tend to occur in the fall and winter months and recede in the spring and summer)
_____ _____ 88. Diet is poor and tends to be haphazard
_____ _____ 89. Do not exercise
_____ _____ 90. Put myself at risk for brain injuries, by doing such things as not wearing my seat belt, drinking and driving, engaging in high-risk sports, etc.
_____ _____ 91. Live under daily or chronic stress, in my home or work life
_____ _____ 92. Thoughts tend to be negative, worried, or angry
_____ _____ 93. Problems getting at least six to seven hours of sleep at night
_____ _____ 94. Smoke or am exposed to secondhand smoke

_____ _____ 95. Drink or consume more than two cups of coffee, tea, or dark sodas a day

_____ _____ 96. Use aspartame and/or MSG

_____ _____ 97. Spends time around environmental toxins, such as paint fumes, hair or nail salon fumes, or pesticides

_____ _____ 98. Spend more than one hour a day watching TV

_____ _____ 99. Spend more than one hour a day playing video games

_____ _____ 100. Outside of work time, spend more than one hour a day on the computer

_____ _____ 101. Consume more than three normal-size drinks of alcohol a week

_____ _____ 102. Struggle with addictions for food, drugs, or behaviors

_____ _____ 103. Struggle with unhealthy cravings, either for food, alcohol, or drugs

_____ _____ 104. Energy is low

Answer "Yes" or "No"

_____ _____ 105. My brain needs help to recover from a brain injury, stroke, drug abuse, moderate to heavy alcohol usage, environmental toxins

UNCHAIN YOUR BRAIN
MASTER QUESTIONNAIRE

Answer Key

Place the number of questions you, or a significant other, answered "3" or "4" in the space provided.

_____ 1 – 10 Prefrontal cortex (PFC) problems, read more about PFC on page 274.

_____ 11 – 20 Anterior cingulate gyrus (ACG) problems, read more about ACG on page 275.

_____ 21 – 30 Deep limbic system (DLS) problems, read more about DLS on page 276.

_____ 31 – 40 Basal ganglia (BG) problems, read more about BG on page 277.

_____ 41 – 50 Temporal lobe (TL) problems, read more about TL on pages 278 – 279.

_____ 51 – 60 Cerebellum problems, read more about Cerebellum on page 280.

_____ 61 – 70 Memory Problems. Consider Dr. Amen's Nutraceutical Solutions Brain & Memory Power Solution

For the six brain systems above and memory problems, find below the likelihood that a problem exists. If there is a potential problem see the corresponding section of the book or the following summary sheets.

5 questions = Highly probable
3 questions = Probable
1-2 questions = May be possible

_____ 71 Insomnia.

_____ 72 – 74 Sleep apnea. If you answered one or more of these questions with a score of "3" or "4" you may have sleep apnea. Sleep apnea occurs when people stop breathing multiple times during the night. It causes significant oxygen deprivation for the brain and people often feel tired and depressed. This condition is best evaluated by a sleep study in a specialized sleep laboratory. Treating sleep apnea often makes a positive difference in mood and energy. If you suspect a problem talk to your physician.

_____ 75 – 78 Hypoglycemia. If you answered three or more questions with a score of "3" or "4" low blood sugar states should be evaluated by your physician. Low blood sugar or hypoglycemia can cause symptoms of anxiety and lethargy. Eating four to five small meals a day, as well as eliminating most of the simple sugars in your diet (such as sugar, bread, pasta, potatoes, and rice) can be very helpful to balance your mood and anxiety levels.

_____ 79 – 85 Scotopic Sensitivity Syndrome. If you answered three or more questions with a score of "3" or "4" you may have Scotopic Sensitivity Syndrome (SSS). SSS occurs when the brain is overly sensitive to certain colors of light. This can cause headaches, anxiety, depression, problems reading, and depth perception issues. Getting this condition properly diagnosed and treated can make a significant difference for your mental and physical health. To learn more about the diagnosis and treatment of SSS go to www.irlen.com. Most physicians do not know about this disorder, so please do not rely on them for accurate information.

_____ 86 Carbohydrate Cravings. If you answered this question with a score of "3" or "4" carbohydrate cravings may be a problem. Dr. Amen's experience led him to develop Craving Control to help people manage their cravings.

_____ 87 Seasonal Mood Disorder. If you answered this question with a score of "3" or "4" you may have a seasonal mood disorder. Getting outside during daylight hours can be helpful, along with sitting in front of special "full spectrum light therapy" devices for thirty minutes in the morning. See http://www.mayoclinic.com/ health/seasonal-affective-disorder/MH00023 for more information.

_____ 88 – 101 Bad Brain Habit Questions. For these questions add up your total score, not just the ones you answered "3" or "4."

> If you score between 0 – 6 then odds are you have very good brain habits. Congratulations! Keep up the good work.

> If you score between 7 – 12 odds are you are doing well, but you can work to be better.

> If you score between 13 – 20 your brain habits are not good and you are prematurely aging your brain. A better brain awaits you.

> If you score more than 20 you have poor brain habits and it is time to be concerned. A brain makeover may just change your life!

_____ 102. Addiction Issues. If you scored "3" or "4" on this question, a comprehensive addiction program could be very helpful, maybe even lifesaving, for you.

> Type 1 Compulsive Addicts
> If you scored "3" or "4" on this question, plus a score of "3" or more on questions 11 – 20 you are likely to have the compulsive addiction type.

> Type 2 Impulsive Addicts
> If you scored "3" or "4" on this question, plus a score of "3" or more on questions 1-10 you are likely to have the impulsive addiction type.

> Type 3 Impulsive-Compulsive Addicts
> If you scored "3" or "4" on this question, plus a score of "3" or more on both questions 1-10 and 11-20 you are likely to have the impulsive-compulsive addiction type.

Type 4 Sad or Emotional Addicts
If you scored "3" or "4" on this question, plus a score of "3" or more on questions 21 – 30 you are likely to have the sad or emotional addiction type.

Type 5 Anxious Addicts
If you scored "3" or "4" on this question, plus a score of "3" or more on questions 31 – 40 you are likely to have the anxious addiction type.

Type 6 Temporal Lobe Addicts
If you scored "3" or "4" on this question, plus a score of "3" or more on questions 41 – 50 you are likely to have the temporal lobe addiction type.

See Chapter 8: Know Your Type for more information.

_____ 103. Cravings. If you scored "3" or "4" on this question, cravings may be a problem for you and you may benefit from information in Chapter 10: Craving Control or our craving formula Craving Control.

_____ 104. Low Energy. If you scored "3" or "4" on this question, low energy may be a problem for you and you may benefit from our Focus & Energy Optimizer.

Answer "Yes" or "No"

_____ 105. My brain needs help to recover from a brain injury, stroke, drug abuse, moderate to heavy alcohol usage, environmental toxins. If you answered "yes" consider our Brain & Memory Power Boost.

Amen Clinics Quick Reference Summaries

Prefrontal Cortex (PFC)

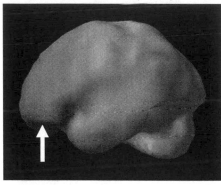

The PFC is the chief executive officer of the brain. It is involved with forethought, judgment and impulse control. Problems in this part of the brain are associated with impulsivity, short attention span, distractibility and difficulties with organization and planning. We have seen a strong correlation with these questions and ADD and impulsive addicts. It may also be associated with certain types of depression, head injuries and toxic exposure.

PFC Functions

Attention
Planning
Follow through
Impulse control
Inhibition
Judgment
Empathy
Learning from
  mistakes

PFC Problems

Inattention
Lack of forethought
Procrastination
Impulsive
Disinhibited
Poor judgment
Lack of empathy
Trouble learning
  from mistakes

PFC Support Supplements

Focus & Energy Optimizer for
  focus and energy support
SAMe Mood & Movement
  Support
Fish oil—*Omega-3 Power*

PFC Meds

For ADD—stimulants, such as
  Adderall or Ritalin
For Depression—Wellbutrin
For Low Energy—Provigil

Some Conditions Affecting the PFC

ADHD
Brain trauma
Schizophrenia
Antisocial
  personality

Depression
Dementia
Conduct disorders
Borderline
  personality

Stimulant addictions, such as to cocaine, methamphetamine, nicotine, or caffeine

Amen Clinics Quick Reference Summaries

Anterior Cingulate Gyrus (ACG)

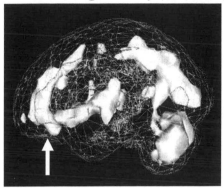

The ACG is the brain's gear shifter. It helps us shift our attention from task to task and idea to idea. It is involved with cognitive flexibility, going with the flow, cooperation and error detection. High scores on this checklist are associated with problems shifting attention which may be manifested by cognitive inflexibility, obsessive thoughts, compulsive behaviors, excessive worrying, being argumentative or oppositional, and "getting stuck" on certain thoughts or actions. Compulsive addicts tend to have too much activity here.

ACG Functions

Brain's gear shifter
Cognitive flexibility
Cooperation
Go from idea to idea
See options
Go with the flow
Error detection

ACG Problems

Gets stuck
Inflexible, worries
Holds grudges
Obsesses
Compulsions
Argumentative
Sees many errors
Oppositional

ACG Support Supplements

Serotonin Mood Support for mood and flexibility support
Fish oil—*Omega-3 Power*

ACG Meds

For Worry, Anxiety and Depression—SSRIs, such as Lexapro, Paxil, Zoloft, Celexa, Prozac, and Luvox

Some Conditions Affecting the ACG

Anxiety disorders   OCD
Eating disorders   PTSD
Chronic pain   PMS
Oppositional   Addictions
    defiant disorder

Compulsive addictions to alcohol and carbohydrates tend to fit this type

Amen Clinics Quick Reference Summaries

Deep Limbic System (DLS)

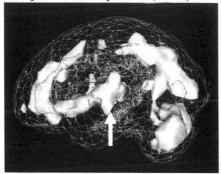

About the size of a walnut, the deep limbic system is involved in setting a person's emotional tone. When the DLS is less active, there is generally a positive, more hopeful state of mind. When it is heated up, or overactive, negativity can take over. Due to this emotional shading, the DLS provides the filter through which you interpret the events of the day; it tags or colors events, depending on the emotional state of mind. The DLS also affects motivation and drive. Overactivity in this area is associated with sadness and mood issues. The DLS also directly processes the sense of smell. Because your sense of smell goes directly to the deep limbic system, it is easy to see why smells can have such a powerful impact on our states of feeling. The problems in the DLS are associated with depression and negativity along with low motivation, libido, and energy.

DLS Functions
Mood control
Charged memories
Motivation
Sets emotional tone
Bonding
Sense of smell
Libido

DLS Problems
Depression
Negative, irritable
Low motivation
Negative, blame
Social isolation
Low self-esteem
Low libido
Decreased interest
Worthlessness
Hopelessness
Mood cycles

DLS Support Supplements
*SAMe Mood & Movement
 Support*
Fish oil—*Omega-3 Power*

DLS Meds
For Depression—
 antidepressants, such as
 Wellbutrin, Effexor or
 Cymbalta; SSRIs (if high
 ACG also present);
 anticonvulsants or lithium
 for cyclic mood changes

Some Conditions Affecting the DLS
Depression
Pain syndromes
Cyclic mood
 disorders

Sad addictions such as to alcohol or opiates

276

Amen Clinics Quick Reference Summaries

Basal Ganglia (BG)

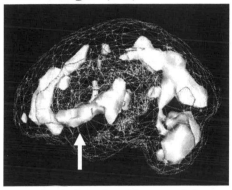

The BG helps set the brain's idle or anxiety level. Increased activity in this part of the brain is often associated with anxiety (left-sided problems are often associated with irritability, right-sided problems more often associated with inwardly directed anxiety). We have seen relaxation therapies, such as biofeedback and hypnosis, and cognitive therapies help calm this part of the brain. If clinically indicated, too much activity here may be helped by calming supplements such as GABA, lemon balm, kava kava, or valerian, or medications, such as buspirone. Sometimes, anti-seizure medications can also be helpful.

BG Functions

Sense of calm
Sets anxiety level
Integrate thoughts
   and feelings
Motor muscle
   movements

BG Problems

Tension, nervousness
Anxiety/panic
Conflict avoidance
Predicting the worst
Tics
Multiple physical
   complaints

BG Support Supplements

For calming support
   GABA Calming Support,
   valerian, kava kava,
   theanine
Fish oil—Omega-3 Power

BG Meds

For Anxiety—Buspar,
   anti-seizure meds, some
   blood pressure meds,
   such as propranolol may
   help

Some Conditions Affecting the BG

Anxiety disorders   OCD
Panic disorders   PTSD
Tourette's syndrome

Anxious addictions to alcohol, marijuana and benzos tend to fit this type

Amen Clinics Quick Reference Summaries

Temporal Lobes (TLs)

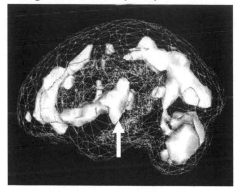

The temporal lobes, underneath your temples and behind your eyes, are involved with language (hearing and reading), reading social cues, short-term memory, getting memories into long-term storage, processing music and tone of voice, and mood stability.

They also help with recognizing objects by sight and naming them. It is called the "What Pathway" in the brain, as it is involved with recognition and naming objects and faces. In addition, the temporal lobes, especially on the right side, have been implicated in spiritual experience and insight. Experiments that stimulate the right temporal lobe have demonstrated increased religious or spiritual experiences, such as feeling God's presence.

Trouble in the temporal lobes leads to both short- and long-term memory problems, reading difficulties, trouble finding the right words in conversation, trouble reading social cues, mood instability, and sometimes religious or moral preoccupation or perhaps a lack of spiritual sensitivity. The temporal lobes, especially on the left side, have been associated with temper problems. Abnormal (high or low) activity in this part of the brain is often due to a deficiency in the neurotransmitter GABA and balancing it through supplements or medications is often helpful.

Amen Clinics Quick Reference Summaries

Temporal Lobes (TLs) continued …

TL Functions	TL Problems
Language	Language problems
Memory	Memory problems
Retrieval of words	Word finding problems
Reading	Dyslexia
Mood stability	Mood instability
Recognize words	Anxiety for no reason
Read social cues	Trouble with social cues
Rhythm	Dark thoughts
Temper control	Aggression
Spiritual experience	Learning problems
	Illusions
	Excess religious ideas

Some Conditions Affecting the TLs

Head injury	Dissociation
Anxiety	Temporal epilepsy
Amnesia	Serious depression
Dyslexia	Dark or suicidal thoughts
Religiosity	

Temporal lobe addictions, such as to alcohol, marijuana, benzos

TL Support Supplements
GABA Calming Support for calming support
Brain & Memory Power Boost for memory support
Fish oil—*Omega-3 Power*

TL Meds
For Mood Stability, Irritability and Anxiety—anti-seizure medications, such as Depakote, Neurontin, Tegretol, and Lamictal

For Memory—memory enhancing medications for more serious memory problems, such as Namenda, Aricept, Exelon, or Reminyl

Amen Clinics Quick Reference Summaries

Cerebellum (CB)

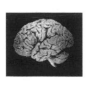 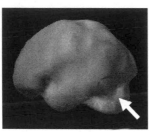 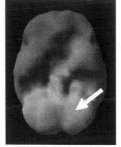 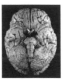

left side surface view   underside surface view

CB Functions
Motor control
Posture, gait
Executive function, connects to
  PFC
Speed of cognitive integration
  (like clock speed of computer)

CB Problems
Gait/coordination problems
Slowed thinking
Slowed speech
Impulsivity
Poor conditioned learning

Some Conditions Affecting CB
Trauma
Alcohol abuse
Autism, Asperger's, ADHD

Cerebellar problems can result from
  various addictions, especially
  alcohol

CB Treatments
Prevention of brain injury
Stop alcohol use or other toxic
  exposure
Occupational therapy
Maximize brain nutrition
Hyperbaric oxygen therapy
Interactive Metronome
Coordination exercises such as
  dance or table tennis

The cerebellum is usually the most active part of the brain and is usually symmetrical in appearance. When it is low in activity it has been associated with ADD, autism, brain trauma, toxic exposure, and coordination and learning problems.

Appendix B

UNCHAIN YOUR BRAIN FROM SPECIFIC ADDICTIONS

What do specific types of substances and behaviors really do to your brain? And how do they affect your mental performance? On the following pages, you will find the answers to these questions. In addition, you will discover common street names for addictive substances, but be aware that slang names change constantly and vary by region.

It's important to understand that street names are more than just a way for people in the drug culture to communicate without letting non-druggies know what they're talking about. Slang is actually a marketing technique that pushers use to entice more people to buy their products. For example, an extremely potent variation of marijuana is sold as "stoner crack." The "stoner" part of the name appeals to potheads who are looking for a high from marijuana. By adding "crack" to the street name, it also draws in users of crack cocaine, thereby doubling the market for the drug. Street names are a tool to manipulate buyers.

In this section, you will also discover proven methods for the treatment of addiction, and information on where to get more specific help. Note that when multiple substances or behaviors are involved, the harmful effects are compounded and treatment may require combination therapies.

No matter what type of substance or behavior has you in its clutches, the therapies that have already been discussed in this book can be helpful:

- Know your motivation (use the One-Page Miracle to define your goals)

- Get the right evaluation (look at the four pillars: bio-psycho-social-spiritual)
- Know your brain type (take the Unchain Your Brain Master Questionnaire)
- Love your brain
- Protect your brain
- Exercise
- Meditate
- Eat a brain healthy diet (find recipes on our website or in the *Change Your Brain, Change Your Body Cookbook*)
- Get adequate sleep
- Get control of your cravings
- Keep your blood sugar balanced
- Give your brain a mental workout
- Practice ANT therapy
- Use stress-management techniques
- Plan how to overcome barriers to brain health
- Take omega-3 fatty acid supplements and other natural supplements for your brain type
- Get your family involved in your recovery

In addition, residential treatment programs, 12-Step programs, psychotherapy, and support groups can be effective ways to combat any type of addiction and are highly recommended if you are having a problem. See the following pages in this section for specifics on how to treat addictions to the following:

- Downers (alcohol, prescription sedatives)
- Psychostimulants (cocaine, methamphetamine, prescription stimulants)
- Opiates (heroin, prescription painkillers)
- Marijuana
- LSD
- Inhalants
- Gambling
- Food addiction
- Sex addiction

- Smoking
- Caffeine

DOWNERS

Alcohol, prescription sedatives
(benzodiazipines like Valium, Xanax, etc.)

Alcohol: beast, booze, brew, firewater, giggle juice, hooch, juice, junkst, moonshine, red-eye

Sedatives: bluebirds, dolls, downie, golf balls, goofers, idiot pills, mother's little helper, V

More than 17 million adults in the U.S. have a drinking problem. About 48 million people have used prescription drugs, such as Valium and Xanax, to get high with about 2,500 teens trying them for recreational use for the first time every day.

What it does to the brain and mental performance:
- Affects coordination centers of the brain (cerebellum) causing motor control problems
- Disrupts the growth of new brain cells
- Affects the hypothalamus causing problems with sexual performance
- Affects the brain stem (medulla), which regulates bodily functions like breathing and heart rate, causing sleepiness, unconsciousness, or death
- Enhances the effects of the neurotransmitter GABA causing sluggishness
- Depresses the central nervous system
- Shrinks the size of the brain
- Raises the risk for dementia
- Associated with depression
- Mental confusion
- Memory and learning problems
- Blackouts and dizziness

What science says works:

For alcohol:
- Eliminate sugar from diet, which can trigger carvings
- N-acetyl-cysteine, 1,200 mg twice a day to help with alcohol cravings
- 12-Step programs
- Neurofeedback to help calm the brain
- Yoga has some positive evidence
- Medical evaluations to help prevent and treat withdrawal symptoms
- Medications depending on your type:
  o Disulfiram, which makes you sick if you drink
  o Acamprosate and naltrexone decrease the buzz from drinking
  o Anticonvulsants to diminish anxiety causing drinking
  o Serotonergic antidepressants for the compulsive drinker
  o The serotonergic antidepressant sertraline was found to be twice as effective in producing abstinence from alcohol when combined with naltrexone compared to placebo.

For prescription sedatives:
- Same as above
- Taper off the drug slowly to minimize withdrawal symptoms
- Medications: Phenobarbital, anticonvulsants

Where to go for help:
Alcoholics Anonymous
www.aa.org

SAMHSA substance abuse treatment facility locator
http://dasis3.samhsa.gov/

PSYCHOSTIMULANTS

Cocaine, methamphetamine, prescription stimulants* (Ritalin, Adderall) in abuse dosages

Cocaine: blow, Bolivian marching powder, coke, crack, flake, happy dust, nose candy, snow

Methamphetamine: chalk, crystal meth, fast, glass, ice, meth, poor man's coke, rock, speed

Prescription stimulants: addies, rits, vitamin R, west coast, uppers

* In appropriate dosages for the right reasons, prescription stimulants can be extremely beneficial for people. Here we are describing inappropriate, recreational use.

Cocaine and methamphetamine are both highly addictive, potent stimulants. Every day, about 2,000 people try cocaine for the first time. In one state, 92.9 percent of violent crimes are attributed to the use of methamphetamine.

What it does to the brain and mental performance:
- Constricts blood vessels in the brain impairing overall brain function
- Marked increases in dopamine
- Impaired memory and learning
- Decreased cognitive flexibility
- Problems with decision-making and planning
- Paranoia
- Aggression
- Obsession
- Anxiety and depression
- Insomnia
- Confusion
- Delusions (the sensation of bugs crawling underneath the skin—meth only)
- Hyperthermia

285

- Stroke
- Tremors and Parkinson's disease-like movement disorders

What science says works:

For all stimulants:
- Find healthy ways to boost energy (Focus & Energy Optimizer)

For cocaine and Meth:
- N-acetyl-cysteine (found in Craving Control)
- Acupuncture
- Transcranial magnetic stimulation
- Aversion therapy
- Medications: antidepressants like Wellbutrin, dopamine agonists (anti-Parkinson's agents), and disulfiram
- If ADD is diagnosed, treatment with prescription stimulants can reduce cocaine cravings

Where to go for help:
Cocaine Anonymous
www.ca.org

OPIATES

Heroin, prescription painkillers (OxyContin, Vicodin, Percodan)

Heroin: big H, black pearl, black tar, brain damage, brown sugar, horse, ska, skag, smack

OxyContin: 40, 80, OCs, hillbilly heroin, kicker, ox, oxy, oxycotton

Heroin is one of the most highly addictive drugs and is one of the worst substances for brain health based on the brain scans I have seen. Nonmedical use of prescription painkillers has skyrocketed. In 2008, 15.2 million Americans age twelve and older had taken a prescription painkiller, tranquilizer, sedative, or stimulant for nonmedical reasons at least once in the past year prior.

What it does to the brain and mental performance:
- It is converted to morphine and binds to the opioid receptors in the brain
- Depresses central nervous system, decreasing breathing rate and heart rate
- With overdose, breathing can stop, causing death
- Reduces anxiety
- Reduces cognitive function
- Slows reaction time
- Impairs memory
- Induces drowsiness

What science says works:
- Acupuncture
- Motivational enhancement strategies
- Phased treatment programs
- Medications: naloxone, naltrexone, buprenorphine, methadone, LAAM, clonidine

Where to go for help:
SAMHSA's National Clearinghouse for Alcohol and Drug Information
800-729-6686

MARIJUANA

420, blunt, bud, cheeba, doobie, ganja, giggle weed, J, herb, Mary Jane, pot

Marijuana is the most commonly used illegal drug, with more than 100 million Americans admitting they have tried it at least once in their lifetime.

What it does to the brain and mental performance:
- Impairs short-term memory

- Learning problems
- Attention problems
- Lack of focus
- Lack of coordination
- Increases risk for psychosis

What science says works:
- Psychosocial therapy
- Drug testing with consequences
- Medications: so far, research has not shown any medications to be helpful for the treatment of marijuana addiction, treatment needs to be targeted to a specific person's type of brain

Where to go for help:
Marijuana Anonymous
www.marijuana-anonymous.org/

LSD

acid, crystal tea, dots, orange haze, rainbow, snowmen, sugar cubes, sunshine

More than 23 million say they have tried LSD.

What it does to the brain and mental performance:
- Acts on serotonin receptors
- Distorts sensory perception
- Long-term memory loss and learning problems
- Dizziness
- Numbness or tremors
- Psychosis
- Flashbacks
- Mania
- Depression
- Hallucinations

What science says works:
- Psychosocial interventions
- Medications: sertraline, naltrexone, clonidine, or benzo-diazepines can be helpful in the treatment of flashbacks

Where to go for help:
SAMHSA substance abuse treatment facility locator
http://dasis3.samhsa.gov/

INHALANTS

hippie crack, huff, moon gas, poor man's pot, Satan's secret, spray, Texas shoeshine, whippets

After looking at more than 57,000 brain scans, I have found that inhalants are the worst drug of abuse for brain function. The brains of inhalant abusers look like Swiss cheese. More than 17 percent of drug-using American adolescents say they got their start by sniffing common household products, such as glue, nail polish remover, paint thinner, and hair sprays.

What it does to the brain and mental performance:
- Affects the brain much faster than many other substances
- Damages the protective myelin coating that surrounds neurons causing cell death
- Affects the cerebellum, causing loss of coordination and balance and slurred speech
- Disrupts new cell growth in the brain's memory centers (hippocampus)
- Smaller gray matter volume
- Chronic use causes tremors and uncontrollable shaking
- Cognitive impairment
- Depression
- Violent behavior
- Personality changes
- Memory loss
- Hallucinations
- Learning problems

What science says works:
- Psychosocial therapy, such as cognitive behavioral therapy
- Motivational enhancement therapy
- Medications: research has not shown any medications to be helpful for the treatment of inhalant addiction

Where to go for help:
SAMHSA substance abuse treatment facility locator
http://dasis3.samhsa.gov/

GAMBLING

action, buck, chalk player, dime bet, hedging, juice, laying the points, sharp, square, wise guy

About 6 to 8 million Americans are either pathological or problem gamblers.

What it does to the brain and mental performance:
- Winning greatly increases activity in the brain's reward system and boosts dopamine
- Almost winning creates the same effect

What science says works:
- N-acetyl-cysteine (found in Craving Control)
- Put someone else in charge of your finances
- Cut up credit cards and ATM cards
- Carry only small amounts of cash
- Use blocking software to block access to any gambling sites on your computer
- Avoid tempting environments

Where to go for help:
National Council on Problem Gambling
800-522-4700

Gamblers Anonymous

www.gamblersanonymous.org

FOOD ADDICTION

binge, eat like a horse, gorge, pig out, stuff oneself, wolf down

Two-thirds of American adults are overweight or obese and more than one-third of children and teens are either currently overweight or at risk of becoming overweight.

What it does to the brain and mental performance:
- Sugar and fat act on the morphine or heroin centers of the brain
- Releases excessive dopamine
- Obesity and overweight shrink and prematurely age the brain
- Reduced gray matter volume
- Increases risk for Alzheimer's disease and dementia
- Increases cognitive impairment
- Depression
- Raises the risk for stroke

What science says works:
- Balance hormones
- Optimize vitamin D levels
- Keep track of daily calorie intake
- Alpha-lipoic acid (found in Craving Control)
- Chromium (found in Craving Control)

Where to go for help:
Dr. Amen's Change Your Brain, Change Your Body website
www.amenclinics.com/cybcyb

SEX ADDICTION

too many terms to list...

Sex addiction is associated with high risk behavior and can include voyeurism, exhibitionism, compulsive masturbation, multiple affairs, many one-night stands, computer pornography, cybersex, and even molestation. Most sex addicts are not sex offenders.

What it does to the brain and mental performance:
- Acts on the brain's reward center
- Releases excessive dopamine
- Boosts serotonin
- Associated with depression
- Suicidal thoughts
- Low self-esteem
- Anxiety

What science says works:
- Couples counseling
- Use blocking software to block Internet pornography and cybersex sites on your computer
- Motivational enhancement therapy
- Medications: naltrexone and serotonin-enhancing anti-depressants (SSRIs)

Where to go for help:
Sex Addicts Anonymous
www.saa-recovery.org
800-477-8191

SMOKING

cancer sticks, cig, coffin nail, smokes

More than an estimated 46 million Americans are smokers, and approximately 4,000 adolescents start smoking every day. The leading cause of death among recovering alcoholics is tobacco-related illness so don't start smoking as a way to help you quit drinking.

What it does to the brain and mental performance:
- Restricts blood flow to the brain
- Binds to receptors for acetycholine, which is involved in learning and memory, muscle function, energy level, heart rate, and respiration
- Raises dopamine levels
- Memory and learning problems

What science says works:
- Hypnosis (Dr. Amen's Stop Smoking Now—Through Hypnosis mp3)
- Keeping track of the number of cigarettes smoked each day
- Have gum, toothpicks, or fresh-cut veggies available for times when you have cravings
- Keep your hands busy with a hobby like knitting or sewing
- Nicotine replacement (patches, gum, lozenges, nasal spray, inhalers)
- Medications: varenicline, nortriptyline, clonidine, and the antidepressants buproprion and Wellbutrin

Where to go for help:
Nicotine Anonymous
www.nicotine-anonymous.org
877-879-6422

American Cancer Society
www.cancer.org
800-227-2345

CAFFEINE

Brew, cuppa, go juice, java, jet fuel, joe, mojo, mud

When we think of caffeine, most of us think of coffee, but caffeine can also be found in tea, energy drinks, sodas, and chocolate.

What it does to the brain and mental performance:
- Restricts blood flow to the brain
- Dehydrates the brain
- Fools the brain into thinking it does not need sleep
- Addictive
- Boosts the stress hormone cortisol

What science says works:
- Taper off consumption to minimize withdrawal symptoms like headache and fatigue
- Consider switching to green tea or decaf
- Drink plenty of water
- Find healthy ways to boost energy (Focus & Energy Optimizer)
- Medication: when treating withdrawal-related headaches, beware that many over-the-counter headache remedies include caffeine as an ingredient

Where to go for help:
You're on your own here, so ask friends and family for support.

Appendix C

CREATING BRAIN HEALTHY ADDICTION TREATMENT PROGRAMS

Both David and I believe it is critical to change the ways addiction treatment is done around the world to include a brain healthy component. Creating brain healthy treatment programs can enhance our ability to navigate the bumpy road to recovery and maintenance. It gives participants the tools they need to create a brain healthy life, which will encourage lifelong sobriety, minimize cravings, and help prevent relapse.

The value of a brain healthy addiction treatment program goes beyond patient success. It is equally important for executives and staff members to understand and live by these principles so treatment centers can be the best they can be. When the employees live a brain healthy life, it means they will be more energetic, more thoughtful, more compassionate, and more successful. This makes them better counselors, nurses, therapists, nutritionists, and managers, which in turn, enhances the treatment programs and increases their effectiveness.

The program recommendations here are based on my experiences and research as a neuroscientist, psychiatrist, and brain imaging specialist, as well as David's vast experience in the addiction field. The following guidelines will help you create a brain healthy addiction treatment program.

1. Do a Complete Evaluation

Perform a comprehensive evaluation of all patients and have staff members conduct an inventory of their own brain health.

- Use the "Unchain Your Brain Master Questionnaire" to determine each patient's brain type, or use SPECT brain imaging for a clearer picture of each patient's brain. Sierra Tucson, a world-class treatment center, now has a SPECT brain imaging camera in their facility, and they send the brain scans to the Amen Clinics for interpretation as a way to better diagnose and treat their patients. (See Case Study: SPECT Brain Imaging at Sierra Tucson later in this section.)

- Take a detailed patient history that includes all four pillars of addiction and healing: biological, psychological, social, and spiritual.

- Test patients' important health numbers. It is critical to know if vitamin deficiencies, hormonal imbalances, or other physical problems may be contributing to their addiction. See Chapter 7: Get the Right Evaluation for a list of tests to perform.

2. Do Not Take a Cookie-Cutter Approach to Treatment

When it comes to treatment, one size does NOT fit all. Treat each patient as an individual based on their specific needs, brain type, gender, and health of their brain. Consider creating specialized treatment tracks for males and females and for different age groups.

- *Adolescents:* Compared to adults, adolescents have higher incidences of dual diagnosis and developmental differences. Because of this young people need a different approach than adults and can benefit from programs that last ninety days rather than the traditional twenty-eight-day program. Because young brains are still developing, adolescents may not yet be hardwired to have the ability to exercise self-control so treatment programs need to be highly structured with clear rules for behavior.

Focus on techniques that strengthen the brain's prefrontal cortex since that area is not fully mature in adolescents. For example, place an emphasis on goal-setting by using the One-Page Miracle, make physical exercise mandatory, and have them practice self-control. Plus, young people often lack the basic life skills they need to make brain healthy choices in life so offer classes or counseling in this area.

- *Seniors:* Older patients who have frontal lobe dementia need special care. Getting a proper diagnosis from an expert in the field of age-related memory loss is the first step. Treating the dementia is critical and may require medication. Focusing on memory-boosting activities can be beneficial for this group.

- *Women:* Female patients may have hormonal imbalances that contribute to addiction and are more likely to have experienced psychosocial trauma or to have an eating disorder. Checking and balancing hormones is key. In addition, therapy for past traumas and education on nutrition are important.

- *Men:* Male patients tend to have a higher incidence of brain trauma that must be diagnosed and treated.

3. Love Your Brain

Provide education to staff, patients, and patients' family members about the brain, how it relates to addiction, and how it is the control and command center of their life. Offer a series of classes on brain health and help the people in your treatment program develop brain envy. Show brain scans of healthy brains and addicted brains for comparison. Then show before-and-after brain scans that prove that by adopting brain healthy habits, you can change your brain and change your life.

- Show the Change Your Brain, Change Your Life DVD and the Which Brain Do You Want DVD.

- Display our posters, "My Brain Is Involved With" and "Which Brain Do You Want" in areas where patients and staff can see them.

- Consider teaching my "Making A Good Brain Great Curriculum," a twelve-session course targeted toward teaching people how to love and care for their brains.

4. Protect Your Brain

- Help protect the brains of your staff and patients from brain injuries. Encourage them to wear helmets whenever participating in high-risk activities like bicycling or skateboarding. Do not let patients hit soccer balls with their heads or engage in any contact sports in your facility.

- Protect them from toxins like cigarette smoke. Smoking reduces blood flow to the brain and lowers brain function, which increases the risk of relapse. For optimal brain recovery, adopt a no-smoking policy for staff and patients. Likewise, protect them from any environmental toxins and make sure your facility is free from mold.

- Limit caffeinated beverages because caffeine constricts blood flow and dehydrates the brain, which may lead to impaired judgment and reduced brain function.

5. Feed Your Brain

- Make a commitment to serve brain healthy foods that enhance the recovery process. Focus on lean protein, low-glycemic/high-fiber carbohydrates, and healthy fats, especially omega-3 fatty acids. If you need help coming up with brain healthy recipes and menus, pick up a copy of the

Change Your Brain, Change Your Body Cookbook, which includes more than sixty brain-boosting recipes.

- If your treatment facility has the space available, plant a vegetable and/or herb garden and use those foods in the meals you serve. Have patients tend the garden as a therapeutic technique to help change their relationship with food and to help them learn to care for something other than themselves.

- Eliminate junk food, sodas, and other sugary beverages from the premises.

- Provide patients with the appropriate brain healthy supplements, including a multiple vitamin and fish oil for all patients, and others based on their brain type.

- Keep a copy of the following list of the fifty best brain foods in the kitchen, dining areas, and employee break room so everyone can become familiar with foods that enhance the brain.

50 Best Brain Foods

Almonds, raw	*Limes*
Almond milk, unsweetened	*Oats*
Apples	*Olives*
Asparagus	*Olive oil*
Avocados	*Oranges*
Bananas	*Peaches*
Beans (black, pinto, garbanzo)	*Peas*
Bell peppers (all colors)	*Plums*
Beets	*Pomegranates*
Blackberries	*Raspberries*
Blueberries	*Red grapes*
Broccoli	*Soybeans*
Brussels sprouts	*Spinach*
Carrots	*Strawberries*

Cheese, low fat	*Tea, green*
Cherries	*Tofu*
Chicken, skinless	*Tomatoes*
Cranberries	*Tuna*
Egg whites, DHA enriched	*Turkey, skinless*
Grapefruit	*Walnuts*
Herring	*Water*
Honeydew	*Whole wheat*
Kiwi	*Wild salmon*
Lemons	*Yams and sweet potatoes*
Lentils	*Yogurt, unsweetened*

Here are a few more nutrition dos and don'ts:

- Don't let employees have candy on their desks.
- Don't bring in (or allow the pharmaceutical company reps to bring in) doughnuts, bagels, or pastries for the break room or for meetings.
- Don't serve sodas or high-sugar drinks at meetings.
- Don't have vending machines stocked with candy and junk food on the premises.
- Do encourage employees who like to share food to have a bowl of fruit or nuts on their desks.
- Do serve fruit, raw veggies, nuts, nonfat or low-fat cheese, and water at meetings.
- Do have caffeine-free herbal teas and decaffeinated teas available.

6. Rest Your Brain

- Set a regular sleep schedule seven days a week in your facility and aim for seven to eight hours of sleep for adults and eight to nine hours for teens.

- Eliminate anything that interferes with sleep, such as caffeine or stimulating behaviors like exercising, scary movies, or video games too close to bedtime. Make it a rule to turn off all computers, phones, and other devices at least one hour before bedtime.

- For people who have trouble sleeping, consider natural sleep aids, such as Restful Sleep.

- For occasional insomnia, you may also want to eat a small carbohydrate-rich, serotonin-enhancing snack in the evening, such as half a peanut butter sandwich or half an apple with a few walnuts.

7. Work Your Brain

- Encourage new learning among patients and staff and strive to learn something new every day.

- Spend fifteen minutes a day learning something new.

- Cross train employees to keep their brain's agile.

- For patients, offer opportunities to learn about art, music, knitting, gardening, cooking, dancing, and more.

- Have crossword puzzles, jigsaw puzzles, and other mentally simulating games available.

8. Exercise Your Brain

- Encourage daily exercise as an integral part of your program for patients and staff.

- Physical activity boosts blood flow, oxygen, and glucose supply to the brain.

- Regular exercise improves cognitive function, strengthens the prefrontal cortex, and decreases cravings.

- Exercise protects the brain against things that hurt it, such as free radicals and high glucose levels.

- The best types of exercises for the brain are those that combine aerobic activity and coordination moves, such as dancing or table tennis (the world's best brain sport).

9. De-stress Your Brain

- Teach brain healthy stress-relief techniques, such as deep breathing, meditation, and self-hypnosis and make them a daily practice.

- Encourage patients and staff to practice gratitude—being thankful for the good things in their lives. As part of your program's daily morning ritual, have patients write down five things they are grateful for. This simple act can have a very powerful effect on mood.

10. Serenade Your Brain

- Make music part of your program by encouraging patients to play musical instruments and sing.

- Play soothing music throughout your facility. Classical music as well as uplifting and calming music can have a beneficial impact on patients.

- Research shows that the songs of the Hawaiian singer Iz (Israel Kamakawiwo'ole) have a tempo similar to resting heart rate, which is about sixty-two beats per minute. Playing his music can calm and regulate heart rate.

11. Kill the ANTs

- Teach patients and staff how to challenge negative thoughts.

- Use the exercises described in Chapter 12: Kill the Addiction ANTs to develop an ANTeater to talk back to negative thoughts.

- Use the four questions of The Work by Byron Katie:
  o Is it true?
  o Can I absolutely know that it is true?
  o How do I feel when I believe that thought?
  o Who would I be without the thought?
  o Turnaround the thought.

12. Treat Brain Problems Early

- Co-occurring conditions are very common in substance abuse.

- Treat them early and aggressively for effectiveness.

- Have an employee assistance plan to help employees who may have a psychiatric or brain issue.

CASE STUDY: NEWPORT ACADEMY

When David was approached to help develop a new residential treatment program for teens in Southern California, he knew he wanted brain health to be part of the program's foundation. From day one, he and the directors created a program based on the brain healthy principles in this book. The result is Newport Academy, a gender-specific, comprehensive program for teens suffering from substance abuse and co-occurring disorders.

At Newport Academy, all patients and their families receive education on the brain and how it relates to addiction and recovery. Using brain scans from the Amen Clinics, David shows images of healthy brains and addicted brains so patients can develop brain envy. Then he shows before-and-after scans that instill patients with hope—hope that their brain can change for the better.

Newport Academy has embraced the power of highly individualized treatment plans rather than taking a one-size-fits-all approach. When patients are difficult to diagnose, Newport Academy orders brain scans from the Amen Clinics. David says, "This has proved invaluable in helping make more accurate diagnoses and treatment plans for some of the patients."

The daily schedule at Newport Academy is also structured to enhance brain health and includes regular exercise, set sleeping schedules, yoga, life skills, goal setting, new learning, nutrition instruction, gardening, spiritual services, family therapy, equine-assisted therapy, and more. This brain healthy approach works. David reports that 85 percent of the adolescents who have completed the Newport Academy program are still sober today.

CASE STUDY: SPECT BRAIN IMAGING AT SIERRA TUCSON

Sierra Tucson has always been at the forefront of addiction treatment. In keeping with its tradition of innovation, the world-renowned center took a giant leap into the future of the treatment of addictions and behavioral disorders when it became the first treatment center to install a SPECT brain imaging camera in its facility in 2009. Patients can be scanned onsite, and Sierra Tucson sends the images to the Amen Clinics for interpretation.

For the treatment specialists, the technology has enhanced their ability to treat their patients effectively. "Now we can actually look at the brain rather than trying to guess at symptom-based cluster categories," says Sierra Tucson's Medical Director Robert Johnson, MD. "It allows us to look at the biological markers that can help with assessment and treatment plans."

After using the technology for more than a year, Dr. Johnson has discovered that brain imaging offers a number of benefits to patients and their families. "Brain scans help to break through denial and the minimization of the impact of substance use," he says. "They are also a great motivating tool. You show a patient a copy of a healthy brain, then you show them their brain and say 'Here's your brain on X,' and ask them 'Which brain do you want?' It does a lot of your work for you."

Dr. Johnson also credits the brain scans for helping patients and their families shift the conversation in addiction from character weakness and lack of willpower to neurobiology. "Particularly with families, it reduces the blame, the criticism, and the black sheep identity. Instead, it creates more patience and compassion," he says. "For the patients, it gives them a clear sense of what the task is, and that is motivating. If it is only about weakness of character, it is a quagmire they don't know how to escape."

So far, Sierra Tucson is scanning about 25-30 percent of patients, with the center's individual doctors determining which patients would benefit most from it. Some doctors wait until a patient has failed to respond to treatment before ordering scans, while others use it to inform their initial assessment and treatment plan.

Sometimes, the results of the scans have been surprising. "It's amazing what you find when you look," says Dr. Johnson. "Things pop up that we wouldn't have been able to pick up otherwise." For example, the brain scans have revealed a much higher than expected incidence of mild traumatic brain injury among patients. One of the common results of those brain injuries is frontal lobe damage, which weakens the ability to say "no" to cravings and strengthens the need for instant gratification, effectively increasing a person's predisposition for addiction and other bad behaviors.

Considering the many benefits of brain imaging, Dr. Johnson expects other treatment centers to begin adding the technology. "This is the direction the field is moving into," he says.

Appendix D

JOURNAL OF PSYCHOACTIVE DRUGS

A Brief History

In the summer of 1967, David E. Smith M.D. launched the *Journal of Psychedelic Drugs* "to compile and disseminate objective information relative to the various types of drugs used in the Haight Ashbury subculture." The *Journal* began as a house organ for the Haight Ashbury Free Medical Clinic of San Francisco but soon found its geographical and topical focus rapidly expanding as the use of a variety of drugs spread throughout the nation and around the world.

By 1974, the *Journal* had successfully expanded to a regular quarterly schedule and had established a professional Editorial Review Board. During the late 1970s, the *Journal* built an international reputation as a respected and authoritative periodical. In 1981 the *Journal* changed its name to the *Journal of Psychoactive Drugs* to better reflect the broad scope of its contents.

Throughout its 40-year history, the *Journal of Psychoactive Drugs* has been on the leading edge of developments in the field of drug use, abuse, and treatment. It has consistently addressed the complex nature of substance use and abuse from a multidisciplinary perspective and has provided in-depth examination of a host of topics, including:

- the disease concept of addiction
- drug use and criminality
- drug use and the elderly
- drug use and sexual behavior
- therapeutic communities

- drug dependence and the family
- women and substance abuse
- professional treatment and the 12-step process
- dual diagnosis
- understanding and preventing relapse
- substance abuse in the workplace

The *Journal* continues to serve both professionals and laypersons alike as an important multidisciplinary forum for critical thinking, analysis, innovation, and evolutionary development in the field of drug use, abuse, and treatment.

Order a subscription to the *Journal of Psychoactive Drugs* today at www.journalofpsychoactivedrugs.com/subscribe.html or use the order form below.

Name_____

Address_____

City/State/ZIP_____

Institution (if applicable)_____

Choose one:
___ U.S. Individual $95
___ Non-U.S. Individual $120
___ U.S. Institution $195
___ Non-U.S. Institution $230

Make check payable to "Journal of Psychoactive Drugs" and mail to:

Haight Ashbury Publications
856 Stanyan St.
San Francisco, CA 94117

REFERENCES AND FURTHER READING

INTRODUCTION

—. 2007. The science of addiction: Drugs, brains, and behavior. *NIH Medline: Plus the Magazine* 2(2):14-17.

Califano, J. 2007. *High Society.* Public Affairs.

Centers for Disease Control and Prevention. 2000. Youth risk behavior surveillance: United States, 1999. *Morbidity and Mortality Weekly Report* 49(SS-5):7.

Danaei, G., E.L. Ding, D. Mozaffarian, et al. 2009. The preventable causes of death in the United States: Comparative risk assessment of dietary, lifestyle, and metabolic factors. *PLoS Medicine* 6(4):e1000058. DOI: 10.1371/journal. pmed.1000 058.

Del Líbano, M., S. Llorens, M. Salanova, et al. 2010. Validity of a brief workaholism scale. *Psicothema* 22(1):143-150.

Hewlett, S.A., and C.B. Luce. 2006. Extreme jobs: The dangerous allure of the 70-hour workweek. *Harvard Business Review* December 2006.

Lenoir, M., F. Serre, L. Cantin, et al. 2007. Intense sweetness surpasses cocaine reward. *PLoS ONE* 2(8):e698. DOI:10.1371/ journal.pone.0000698.

SAMHSA/DAWN. National estimates, drug-related emergency department visits for 2004–2008.

Tjaden, P., and N. Thoennes. 2000. U.S. Department of Justice, NCJ 183781, Full Report of the Prevalence, Incidence, and

Consequences of Intimate Partner Violence Against Women: Findings from the National Violence Against Women Survey.

Waters, H., A. Hyder, Y. Rajkotia, et al. 2004. The economic dimensions of interpersonal violence. Department of Injuries and Violence Prevention, World Health Organization, Geneva.

CHAPTER 1

National Institute on Alcohol Abuse and Alcoholism. 2003. *Assessing Alcohol Problems: A Guide for Clinicians and Researchers, 2d ed.* NIH Pub. No. 03–3745. Washington, DC: U.S. Dept. of Health and Human Services, Public Health Service.

CHAPTER 2

Camargo, E.E. 2001. Brain SPECT in neurology and psychiatry. *Journal of Nuclear Medicine* 42(4):611-623.

Catafau, A.M. 2001. Brain SPECT in clinical practice. Part I: Perfusion. *Journal of Nuclear Medicine* 42(2):259-271.

Vasile, R.G. 1996. Single photon emission computed tomography in psychiatry: Current perspectives. *Harvard Review of Psychiatry* 4(1):27-38.

CHAPTER 3

Holman, B.L., P.A. Carvalho, J. Mendelson, et al. 1991. Brain perfusion is abnormal in cocaine-dependent polydrug users: A study using technetium-99m-HMPAO and SPECT. *Journal of Nuclear Medicine* 32:1206-1210.

Kao, C.H., S.J. Wang, and S.H. Yeh. 1994. Presentation of regional cerebral blood flow in amphetamine abusers by 99Tcm-HMPAO brain SPECT. *Nuclear Medicine Communications* 15:94-98.

Küçük, N.O., E.O. Kiliç, E. Ibis, et al. 2000. Brain SPECT findings in long-term inhalant abuse. *Nuclear Medicine Communications* 21(8):769-773.

Levin, J.M., B.L. Holman, J.H. Mendelson, et al. 1994. Gender differences in cerebral perfusion in cocaine abuse: Technetium-99m-HMPAO SPECT study of drug-abusing women. *Journal of Nuclear Medicine* 35:1902-1909.

Mena, I., R.J. Giombetti, B.L. Miller, et al. 1994. Cerebral blood flow changes with acute cocaine intoxication: Clinical correlations with SPECT, CT, and MRI. *NIDA Research Monograph* 138:161-173.

Mendelson, J.H., B.L. Holman, S.K. Teoh, et al. 1995. Improved regional cerebral blood flow in chronic cocaine polydrug users treated with buprenorphine. *Journal of Nuclear Medicine* 36:1211-1215.

Miller, B.L., I. Mena, R. Giombetti, et al. 1992. Neuropsychiatric effects of cocaine: SPECT measurements. *Journal of Addictive Diseases* 11:47-58.

Ryu, Y.H., J.D. Lee, P.H. Yoon, et al. 1998. Cerebral perfusion im-pairment in a patient with toluene abuse. *Journal of Nuclear Medicine* 39(4):632-3.

Saxena, S., A.L. Brody, J.M. Schwartz, et al. 1998. Neuroimaging and frontal-subcortical circuitry in obsessive-compulsive disorder. *British Journal of Psychiatry Supplement* (35):26-37.

Tumeh, S.S., J.S. Nagel, R.J. English, et al. 1990. Cerebral abnormalities in cocaine abusers: Demonstration by SPECT perfusion brain scintigraphy. *Radiology* 176:821-824.

Volkow, N.D., J.S. Fowler, G.J. Wang, et al. 1993. Decreased dopamine D2 receptor availability is associated with reduced frontal metabolism in cocaine abusers. *Synapse* 14:169-177.

CHAPTER 4

10,000 Kids Publication. 2007. *Crystal Darkness Las Vegas: Meth's Deadly Assault on our Families.*

Baker, R. 2008. "Minn. Jury Awards $8.3 Million in First Mirapex Trial." Andrews Publication August 7, 2008.

Bostwick, J.M., K.A. Hecksel, S.R. Stevens, et al. 2009. Frequency of new-onset pathologic compulsive gambling or hyper-sexuality after drug treatment of idiopathic Parkinson disease. *Mayo Clinic Proceedings* 84(4):310-6.

Crockford, D.N., B. Goodyear, J. Edwards, et al. 2005. Cue-induced brain activity in pathological gamblers. *Biological Psychiatry* 58(10):787-95.

Danaei G., Ding E.L., Mozaffarian D., Taylor B., Rehm J., et al. 2009. The preventable causes of death in the United States: Comparative risk assessment of dietary, lifestyle, and metabolic risk factors. *PLoS Med* 6(4): e1000058; DOI: 10.1371/journal.pmed.1000058.

Gailliot, M.T., and Baumeister, R.F. 2007. The physiology of will-power: linking blood glucose to self-control. *Personality and Social Psychology Review* 11:303. DOI:10.1177/1088868307 303030.

Giladi, N., N. Weitzman, S. Schreiber, et al. 2007. New onset heightened interest or drive for gambling, shopping, eating or sexual activity in patients with Parkinson's disease: The role of dopamine agonist treatment and age at motor symptoms onset. *Journal of Psychopharmacology* 21(5):501-6.

Kessler, D., MD. 2009. *The End of Overeating,* New York: Rodale.

Khaw, K.T., N. Wareham, S. Bingham, et al. 2008. Combined impact of health behaviours and mortality in men and women:

The EPIC-Norfolk prospective population study. *PLoS Medicine* 5(1):e12. doi:10.1371/journal.pmed.0050012.

Liebschutz, J., J.B. Savetsky, R. Saitz, et al. 2002. The relationship between sexual and physical abuse and substance abuse consequences. *Journal of Substance Abuse Treatment* 22(3):121-128.

Mandyam, C.D., R.W. Kotzebue, E.F. Crawford, et al. 2009. Chronic voluntary alcohol consumption produces permanent impairment of hippocampal neurogenesis in adolescent nonhuman primates. Presented at Neuroscience 2009, October 17, 2009.

Munhoz, R.P., G. Fabiani, N. Becker, et al. 2009. Increased frequency and range of sexual behavior in a patient with Parkinson's disease after use of pramipexole: A case report. *The Journal of Sexual Medicine* 6(4):1177-80.

Nestler, E.J. 2009. Transcriptional and epigenetic mechanisms of drug addiction. Presented at Neuroscience 2009, October 21, 2009.

NIDA (National Institute on Drug Abuse), U.S. Department of Health and Human Services/National Institutes of Health. 2008. *Comorbidity: Addiction and Other Mental Illnesses.* NIH Publication #08-5771.

NIDA (National Institute on Drug Abuse), U.S. Department of Health and Human Services/National Institutes of Health. 2007. *Drugs, Brains, and Behavior: The Science of Addiciton.* NIH Publication #07-5605.

Ondo, W.G., and D. Lai. 2008. Predictors of impulsivity and reward seeking behavior with dopamine agonists. *Parkinsonism & Related Disorders* 14(1):28-32.

Paul, C.A., R. Au, L. Fredman, et al. 2008. Association of alcohol consumption with brain volume in the Framingham Study.

Archives of Neurology 65(10):1363-1367. DOI: 10.1001/ archneur.65.10.1363.

Porter, J.N., A.S. Olsen, K. Gurnsey, et al. 2009. Longitudinal studies of cocaine self-administration on cognition in rhesus monkeys. Presented at Neuroscience 2009, October 18, 2009.

Pourcher, E., S. Rémillard, H. Cohen. 2010. Compulsive habits in restless legs syndrome patients under dopaminergic treatment. *Journal of the Neurological Sciences* 290(1-2):52-56.

Riba, J., U.M. Krämer, M. Heldmann, et al. 2008. Dopamine agonist increases risk taking but blunts reward-related brain activity. *PLoS One* 3(6):e2479.

Rohsenow, D.J., J. Howland, and J.T. Arnedt. 2009. Intoxication with bourbon versus vodka: Effects on hangover, sleep, and next-day neurocognitive performance in young adults. *Alcohol, Clinical and Experimental Research* Dec 17 [Epub ahead of print].

Sayette, M.A., J.W. Schooler, and E.D. Reichle. 2009. Out for a smoke: The impact of cigarette craving on zoning out during reading. *Psychological Science* published online before print November 23, 2009. DOI: 10.1177/0956797609354059.

Sharot, T., T. Shiner, A.C. Brown, et al. 2009. Dopamine enhances expectation of pleasure in humans. *Current Biology* 19(24): 2077-2080. DOI: 10.1016/j.cub.2009.10.025.

Stamey, W., and J. Jankovic. 2008. Impulse control disorders and pathological gambling in patients with Parkinson disease. *Neurologist* 14(2):89-99.

Tang, J., and J. Dani. 2009. Dopamine Enables In Vivo Synaptic Plasticity Associated with the Addictive Drug Nicotine. *Neuron* 63(5):673-682.

The Solutions Foundation. It's Tough Being a Teen… Don't Make it Tougher! www.solutions-foundation.org.

VanDellen, M.R., and R.H. Hoyle. 2009. Regulatory accessibility and social influences on state self-control. *Personality and Social Psychology Bulletin Online First* 36(2):251-256. DOI:10.1177/ 0146167209356302

Volkow, N.D., G.J. Wang, F. Telang, et al. 2009. Inverse assoc-iation between BMI and prefrontal metabolic activity in healthy adults. *Obesity* (Silver Spring) 17(1):60-5.

Volkow, N.D. 2009. Addiction and self-control. Presented at Neuroscience 2009, October 19, 2009.

Volkow, N.D., G.J. Wang, J.S. Fowler, et al. 2008. Overlapping neuronal circuits in addiction and obesity: evidence of systems pathology. *Philosophical Transactions of the Royal Society of London, Series B Biological Sciences* 363(1507):3191-200.

Volkow, N.D., G.J. Wang, F. Telang, et al. 2008. Low dopamine striatal D2 receptors are associated with prefrontal metabolism in obese subjects: possible contributing factors. *Neuroimage* 42(4):1537-43.

Volpicelli, J., G. Balaraman, J. Hahn, et al. 1999. The role of uncontrollable trauma in the development of PTSD and alcohol addiction. *Alcohol Research & Health* 23:256-262.

Voon, V., B. Reynolds, C. Brezing, et al. 2009. Impulsive choice and response in dopamine agonist-related impulse control behaviors. *Psychopharmacology* October 20, 2009 [Epub ahead of print].

Wang, G.J., N. Volkow, K. T. Panayotis, et al. 2009. Imaging of brain dopamine pathways: Implications for understanding obesity. *Journal of Addiction Medicine* 3(1):8-18.

Wang, G.J., N.D. Volkow, P.K. Thanos, et al. 2004. Similarity between obesity and drug addiction as assessed by neurofunctional imaging: a concept review. *Journal of Addictive Diseases* 23(3):39-53.

Wang, G.J., N.D. Volkow, and J.S. Fowler. 2002. The role of dopamine in motivation for food in humans: implications for obesity. *Expert Opinion on Therapeutic Targets* 6(5):601-9.

Weintraub, D., A.D. Siderowf, M.N. Potenza, et al. 2006. Association of dopamine agonist use with impulse control disorders in Parkinson disease. *Archive of Neurology* 63(7):969-73.

Wolraich, M.L., C.J. Wibbelsman, T.E. Brown, et al. 2005. Attention-deficit/hyperactivity disorder among adolescents: A review of the diagnosis, treatment, and clinical implications. *Pediatrics* 115:1734-1746.

Zupec-Kania, B., and M.L. Zupanc. 2008. Long-term management of the ketogenic diet: Seizure monitoring, nutrition, and supplementation. *Epiliepsia* 49(Supplement 8):23-26.

CHAPTER 5

Amen, D.G. *Healing ADD*. New York: Berkley Books, 2001.

Armentano, M.E., and R. Sohlkhah. 2003. Co-occurring disorders in adolescents. Chapter in Graham, A.W., T.K. Schultz, M.F. Mayo-Smith, et al. 2003. *Principles of Addiction Medicine, 3rd ed.* Chevy Chase, MD: American Society of Addiction Medicine. 2003.

Berthier, M.L., J. Kulisevsky, A. Gironell, et al. 2001. Obsessive-compulsive disorder and traumatic brain injury: Behavioral, cognitive, and neuroimaging findings. *Neuropsychiatry, Neuropsychology & Behavioral Neurology* 14(1):23-31.

Biederman, J., M.C. Monuteaux, T. Spencer, et al. 2008. Stimulant therapy and risk for subsequent substance use disorders in male adults with ADHD: a naturalistic controlled 10-year follow-up study. *American Journal of Psychiatry* 165:597-603.

Biederman, J., T. Wilens, E. Mick, et al. 1999. Pharmacotherapy of attention-deficit/hyperactivity disorder reduces risk for substance use disorder. *Pediatrics* 104:e20.

Bloom, D.R., H.S. Levin, L. Ewing-Cobbs, et al. 2001. Lifetime and novel psychiatric disorders after pediatric traumatic brain injury. *Journal of the American Academy of Child & Adolescent Psychiatry* 40(5):572-579.

Buydens-Branchey, L., M. Branchey, D.L. McMakin, et al. 2003. Polyunsaturated fatty acid status and relapse vulnerability in cocaine addicts. *Psychiatry Research* 120(1):29-35.

Cappuccio, F. 2006. Obesity in children and adults: sleep deprivation doubles risk. Presented at the 2006 International AC21 Research Festival.

Carpenter, S. 2001. Sleep deprivation may be undermining teen health. *Monitor on Psychology* 32(9).

Christakis, D.A., and M.A. Moreno. 2009. Trapped in the net: Will Internet addiction become a 21st-century epidemic? *Archives of Pediatrics & Adolescent Medicine* 163(10):959-960.

Chung, S., F. Woodward Hopf, H. Nagasaki, et al. 2009. The melanin concentrating hormone system modulates cocaine reward. *Proceedings of the National Academy of Sciences of the USA* 106(16):6772-6777. DOI: 10.1073/pnas.0811331106.

DeSantis, A.D., E.M. Webb, and S.M. Noar. 2008. Illicit use of prescription ADHD medications on a college campus: a multimethodological approach. *Journal of American College Health* 57(3):315-24.

Durmer, J.S., and D.F. Dinges. 2005. Neurocognitive consequences of sleep deprivation. *Seminars in Neurology* 25:117-129.

Forquer, L.M., A.E. Camden, K.M. Gabriau, C.M. Johnson. 2008. Sleep patterns of college students at a public university. *Journal of American College Health* 56(5):563-565.

Froehlich, T.E., B.P. Lanphear, P. Auinger, et al. 2009. Association of tobacco and lead exposures with attention-deficit/hyperactivity disorder. *Pediatrics* 124(6):e1054-63. DOI:10.1542/peds.2009-0738.

Hennessey, K.A., M.D. Stein, C. Rosengard, et al. 2009. Childhood attention deficit hyperactivity disorder, substance use, and adult functioning among incarcerated women. *Journal of Attention Disorders* September 22, 2009 [Epub ahead of print].

Jaffe, H. 2006. "ADD & Abusing Adderall." *Washingtonian.com* January 1, 2006.

Kim, B.N., S.C. Cho, Y. Kim, et al. 2009. Phthalates exposure and attention-deficit/hyperactivity disorder in school-age children. *Biological Psychiatry* 66(10):958-63. DOI: 10.1016/j.biopsych.2009.07.034.

Ko, C.H., J.Y. Yen, C.S. Chen, et al. 2009. Predictive values of psychiatric symptoms for Internet addiction in adolescents: A 2-year prospective study. *Archives of Pediatrics & Adolescent Medicine* 163(10):937-943.

Mannuzza, S., R.G. Klein, N.L. Truon, et al. 2008. Age of methylphenidate treatment initiation in children with ADHD and later substance abuse: Prospective follow-up into adulthood. *American Journal of Psychiatry* 165:604-609.

McCabe, S.E., J.R. Knight, C.J. Teter, et al. 2005. Non-medical use of prescription stimulants among US college students:

Prevalence and correlates from a national survey. *Addiction* 100(1):96-106.

Mick, E. 1998. Adult ADHD increases the risk of substance abuse. Presented at the 1998 annual meeting of the American Academy of Child and Adolescent Psychiatry. *Clinical Psychiatry News* 26(2):5.

NIDA (National Institute on Drug Abuse), U.S. Department of Health and Human Services/National Institutes of Health. 2007. *Drugs, Brains, and Behavior: The Science of Addiciton.* NIH Publication #07-5605.

Nedeltcheva, A., et al. 2009. Exposure to recurrent sleep restriction in the setting of high caloric intake and physical inactivity results in increased insulin resistance and reduced glucose tolerance. *Journal of Clinical Endocrinology & Metabolism* 94(9):3242-3250. DOI: 10.1210/jc.2009-0483.

Nelson, M., and P. Gordon-Larsen. 2006. Physical activity and sedentary behavior patterns are associated with selected adolescent health risk behaviors. *Pediatrics* 117(4):1281-1290.

Owens, J. 2008. Sleep disorders and attention-deficit/hyperactivity disorder. *Current Psychiatry Reports* 10(5):439-444.

Parks, C., National Institute of Environmental Health Sciences. Presentation at American College of Rheumatology annual meeting, Philadelphia, Oct. 17, 2009.

Patel, S., et al. 2006. Association between reduced sleep and weight gain in women. *American Journal of Epidemiology.* 164(10):947-954.

Perello, M., I. Sakata, S. Birnbaum, et al. 2009. Ghrelin increases the rewarding value of high-fat diet in an orexin-dependent manner. *Biological Psychiatry* online December 24, 2009. [Epub ahead of print]. DOI: 10.1016/j.biopsych.2009.10.030.

Roane, B., and D. Taylor. 2008. Adolescent insomnia as a risk factor for early adult depression and substance abuse. *Sleep* 31(10):1351-1356.

Spiegel, K., E. Tasali, R. Leproult, E. Van Cauter. 2009. Effects of poor and short sleep on glucose metabolism and obesity risk. *Nature Reviews Endocrinology* 5(5):253-261.

Sponaugle, M.R. 2009. Anti-aging/longevity medicine reduces the prevalence of alcoholism and drug addiction.

Suh, J.J., D.D. Langleben, R.N. Ehrman, et al. 2009. Low pre-frontal perfusion linked to depression symptoms in methadone-maintained opiate-dependent patients. *Drug and Alcohol Dependence* 99(1-3):11-17.

Taheri, S., L. Lin, D. Austin, T. Young, E. Mignot. 2004. Short sleep duration is associated with reduced leptin, elevated ghrelin, and increased body mass index. *PLoS Med* 1(3):e62.

Teter, C.J., S.E. McCabe, K. LaGrange, et al. 2006. Illicit use of specific prescription stimulants among college students: prevalence, motives, and routes of administration. *Pharmacotherapy* 26(10):1501-10.

Talbot, M. 2009. Brain gain: The underground world of "neuro-enhancing" drugs. *The New Yorker* April 27, 2009.

Uher, R., and J. Treasure. 2005. Brain lesions and eating disorders. *Journal of Neurology, Neurosurgery, & Psychiatry* 76:852-857. DOI:10.1136/jnnp.2004.048819.

Vitiello, B. 2001. Long-term effects of stimulant medications on the brain: Possible relevance to the treatment of attention deficit hyperactivity disorder. *Journal of Child & Adolescent Psychopharmacology* 11:25-34.

Volkow, N.D., and J.M. Swanson. 2008. Does childhood treatment of ADHD with stimulant medication affect substance abuse in adulthood? *American Journal of Psychiatry* 165:553-555.

Walker, R., J.E. Cole, T.K. Logan, et al. 2007. Screening substance abuse treatment clients for traumatic brain injury: Prevalence and characteristics. *Journal of Head Trauma Rehabilitation* 22(6):360-7.

Weyandt, L.L., G. Janusis, K.G. Wilson, et al. 2009. Nonmedical prescription stimulant use among a sample of college students: relationship with psychological variables. *Journal of Attention Disorders* 13(3):284-96.

Yücel, M., and D.I. Lubman. 2007. Neurocognitive and neuro-imaging evidence of behavioural dysregulation in human drug addiction: Implications for diagnosis, treatment and prevention. *Drug and Alcohol Review* 26(1):33-9.

CHAPTER 6

White, K.G., and J. Cameron. 2000. Resistance to change, contrast, and intrinsic motivation. *Behavioral and Brain Sciences* 23:1: 115-116

Williams, B.A., and M.C. Bell. 2000. The uncertain domain of resistance to change. *Behavioral and Brain Sciences* 23:1:116-117

CHAPTER 7

Biederman, J., T. Wilens, E. Mick, et al. 1999. Pharmacotherapy of attention-deficit/hyperactivity disorder reduces risk for substance use disorder. *Pediatrics* 104:e20.

Etchebehere, E.C., F.M. Oliveira, B.J. Amorim, et al. 2010. Brain hypoperfusion in adolescents dependent of multiple drugs. *Arquivos Neuropsiquiatria* 68(2):161-167.

Hennessey, K.A., M.D. Stein, C. Rosengard, et al. 2009. Childhood attention deficit hyperactivity disorder, substance use, and adult functioning among incarcerated women. *Journal of Attention Disorders* September 22, 2009 [Epub ahead of print].

Hibbeln, J.R., T.A. Ferguson, and T.L. Blasbalg. 2006. Omega-3 fatty acid deficiencies in neurodevelopment, aggression and autonomic dysregulation: opportunities for intervention. *International Review of Psychiatry* 18(2):107-118.

Ishizawa, K.T., H. Kumano, A. Sato, et al. 2010. Decreased response inhibition in middle-aged male patients with type 2 diabetes. *BioPsychoSocial Medicine* 4:1. DOI:10.1186/1751-0759-4-1.

Johann, M., G. Bobbe, A. Putzhammer, et al. 2003. Comorbidity of alcohol dependence with attention-deficit hyperactivity disorder: differences in phenotype with increased severity of the substance disorder, but not in genotype (serotonin transporter and 5-hydroxytryptamine-2c receptor). Alcoholism, Clinical and Experimental Research 27(10):1527-1534.

Mannuzza, S., R.G. Klein, N.L. Truon, et al. 2008. Age of methylphenidate treatment initiation in children with ADHD and later substance abuse: Prospective follow-up into adulthood. *American Journal of Psychiatry* 165:604-609.

Mick, E. 1998. Adult ADHD increases the risk of substance abuse. Presented at the 1998 annual meeting of the American Academy of Child and Adolescent Psychiatry. *Clinical Psychiatry News* 26(2):5.

Solomon, A., M. Kivipelto, B. Wolozin, et al. 2009. Midlife serum cholesterol and increased risk of Alzheimer's and vascular dementia three decades later. *Dementia and Geriatric Cognitive Disorders* 28(1):75-80. DOI: 10.1159/000231980.

Volkow, N.D., and J.M. Swanson. 2008. Does childhood treatment of ADHD with stimulant medication affect substance abuse in adulthood? *American Journal of Psychiatry* 165:553-555.

Walker, R., J.E. Cole, T.K. Logan, et al. 2007. Screening substance abuse treatment clients for traumatic brain injury: Prevalence and characteristics. *Journal of Head Trauma Rehabilitation* 22(6):360-7.

Wolraich, M.L., C.J. Wibbelsman, T.E. Brown, et al. 2005. Attention-deficit/hyperactivity disorder among adolescents: A review of the diagnosis, treatment, and clinical implications. *Pediatrics* 115(6):1734-1746.

CHAPTER 8

American Psychiatric Association. 2000. *Diagnostic and Statistical Manual of Mental Disorders*. Washington, DC.

Centers for Disease Control and Prevention. 2006. Behavioral Risk Factor Surveillance System (BRFSS).

Brener, N. D., P.M. McMahon, and C.W. Warren. 1999. Forced sexual intercourse and associated health-risk behaviors among female college students in the United States. *Journal of Consulting and Clinical Psychology* 67(2):252-259.

Breslau, N., G.C. Davis, P. Andreski, et al. 1991. Traumatic events and posttraumatic stress disorder in an urban population of young adults. *Archives of General Psychiatry* 48:216-222.

Kessler, R.C., P. Berglund, O. Demler, et al. 2003. The epidemiology of major depressive disorder: Results from the National Comorbidity Survey Replication (NCS-R). *Journal of the American Medical Association* 289(23):3095-3105.

Kessler, R.C., A. Sonnega, E. Bromet, et al. 1995. Posttraumatic stress disorder in the National Comorbidity Survey. *Archives of General Psychiatry* 52(12):1048-1060.

Newman, M.F., J.L. Kirchner, B. Phillips-Bute, et al. 2001. Longitudinal assessment of neurocognitive function after coronary-artery bypass surgery. *New England Journal of Medicine* 344(6):395–402.

Norris, F. H., J.D. Foster, and D.L. Weishaar. 2002. The epidemiology of sex differences in PTSD across developmental, societal, and research contexts. In R. Kimerling, P. Ouimette & J. Wofle (Eds.), *Gender and PTSD* (pp. 3-42). New York: The Guilford Press.

Pastor, P.N., and C.A. Reuben. 2008. Diagnosed attention deficit hyperactivity disorder and learning disability: United States, 2004–2006. National Center for Health Statistics. *Vital and Health Statistics* 10(237).

Selnes, O.A., R.M. Royall, M.A. Grega, et al. 2001. Cognitive changes 5 years after coronary artery bypass grafting. *Archives of Neurology* 58(4):598–604.

Tjaden, P., and N. Thoennes. 2000. Prevalence and consequences of male-to-female and female-to-male intimate partner violence as measured by the national violence against women survey. *Violence Against Women* 6(2):142-161.

Tolin, D. F., and E.B. Foa. 2002. Gender and PTSD: A cognitive model. In R. Kimerling, P. Ouimette & J. Wolfe (Eds.), *Gender and PTSD* (pp. 76-97). New York: The Guilford Press.

CHAPTER 9

Al'Absi, M., editor. 2006. *Stress and Addiction: Biological and Psychological Mechanisms*. Academic Press.

Alfredson, B.B., J. Risberg, B. Hagberg, et al. 2004. Right temporal lobe activation when listening to emotionally significant music. *Applied Neuropsychology* 11(3):161-166.

Angelo, D.L., H. Tavares, H.M. Bottura, et al. 2009. Physical exercise for pathological gamblers. *Revista Brasileira de Psiquiatria* 31(1):76. DOI: 10.1590/S1516-44462009000100 017.

Brown, R.A., A.M. Abrantes, J.P. Read, et al. 2008. Aerobic exercise for alcohol recovery: Rationale, program description, and preliminary findings. *Behavior Modification* 33(2):220-249.

Cheek, J.M., and L.R. Smith. 1999. Music training and mathematics achievement. *Adolescence* 34(136):759-761.

Hosseini, M., H.A. Alaei, A. Naderi, et al. 2009. Treadmill exercise reduces self-administration of morphine in male rats. *Pathophysiology* 16(1):3-7.

Schellenberg, E.G. 2004. Music lessons enhance IQ. *Psychological Science* 15(8):511-514.

Schmithorst, V.J., and S.K. Holland. 2004. The effect of musical training on the neural correlates of math processing: A functional magnetic resonance imaging study in humans. *Neuroscience Letters* 354(3):193-196.

Schulkind, M.D., L.K. Hennis, and D.C. Rubin. 1999. Music, emotion, and autobiographical memory: They're playing your song. *Memory and Cognition* 27(6):948-955.

Socker, Steven. 1999. Studies link stress and addiction. *NIDA Notes* 14(1).

Taylor, A.H., M.H. Ussher, and G. Faulkner. 2007. The acute effects of exercise on cigarette cravings, withdrawal symptoms, affect and smoking behaviour: A systematic review. *Addiction* 102(4):534-543.

Ussher, M.H., A. Taylor, and G. Faulkner. 2008. Exercise interventions for smoking cessation. *Cochrane Database of*

Systematic Reviews (4):CD002295.

Van Rensburg, K.J., A. Taylor, and T. Hodgson. 2009. The effects of acute exercise on attentional bias towards smoking-related stimuli during temporary abstinence from smoking. *Addiction* 104(11):1910-1917.

Van Rensburg K.J., A. Taylor, T. Hodgson, et al. 2009. Acute exercise modulates cigarette cravings and brain activation in response to smoking-related images: An fMRI study. *Psychopharmacology* (Berl) 203(3):589-598.

Van Rensburg K.J., and A.H. Taylor. 2008. The effects of acute exercise on cognitive functioning and cigarette cravings during temporary abstinence from smoking. *Human Psychopharmacology* 23(3):193-199.

CHAPTER 10

Angelo, D.L., H. Tavares, H.M. Bottura, et al. 2009. Physical exercise for pathological gamblers. *Revista Brasileira de Psiquiatria* 31(1):76. DOI: 10.1590/S1516-44462009000100-017.

Avena, N.M., P. Rada, and B.G. Hoebel. 2009. Sugar and fat bingeing have notable differences in addictive-like behavior. *Journal of Nutrition* 139(3):623-628.

Avena, N.M., P. Rada, and B.G. Hoebel. 2008. Underweight rats have enhanced dopamine release and blunted acetylcholine response in the nucleus accumbens while bingeing on sucrose. *Neuroscience* 156(4):865-871.

Avena, N.M., C.A. Carrillo, L. Needham, et al. 2004. Sugar-dependent rats show enhanced intake of unsweetened ethanol. *Alcohol* 34(2-3):203-209.

Barson, J.R., A.J. Carr, J.E. Soun, et al. 2010. Opioids in the hypothalamic paraventricular nucleus stimulate ethanol intake.

Alcoholism, Clinical and Experimental Research 34(2):214-222.

Berner, L.A., N.M. Avena, and B.G. Hoebel. 2008. Bingeing, self-restriction, and increased body weight in rats with limited access to a sweet-fat diet. *Obesity* (Silver Spring) 16(9):1998-2002.

Bordnick, P.S., H.L. Copp, A. Traylor, et al. 2009. Reactivity to cannabis cues in virtual reality environment. *Journal of Psychoactive Drugs* 41(2):105-112.

Brown, R.A., A.M. Abrantes, J.P. Read, et al. 2008. Aerobic exercise for alcohol recovery: Rationale, program description, and preliminary findings. *Behavior Modification* 33(2):220-249.

Carnicella, S., and D. Ron. 2009. GDNF: A potential target to treat addiction. *Pharmacology & Therapeutics* 122:9-18

Chen, X.S., H. Liu, A.M. Ji, et al. 2009. Effects of sustained-release alpha-lipoic acid tablet on blood lipid, blood sugar and insulin in hyperlipidemic New Zealand rabbits. *Nan Fang Yi Ke Da Xue Xue Bao* 29(4):704-706.

Cummings, B.P., K.L. Stanhope, J.L. Graham, et al. 2010. Dietary fructose accelerates the development of diabetes in UCD-T2DM rats: Amelioration by the antioxidant, {alpha}-lipoic acid. *American Journal of Physiology: Regulatory, Integrative and Comparative Physiology* February 10, 2010. [Epub ahead of print]

Grant, J.E., S.W. Kim, and B.L. Odlaug. 2007. N-acetyl cysteine, a glutamate-modulating agent, in the treatment of pathological gambling: a pilot study. *Biological Psychiatry* 62(6):652-657.

Hosseini, M., H.A. Alaei, A. Naderi, et al. 2009. Treadmill exercise reduces self-administration of morphine in male rats. *Pathophysiology* 16(1):3-7.

Knackstedt, L.A., R.I. Melendez, and P.W. Kalivas. 2010. Ceftria-xone restores glutamate homeostasis and prevents relapse to cocaine seeking. *Biological Psychiatry* 67(1):81-84.

Knackstedt, L.A., S. LaRowe, P. Mardikian, et al. 2009. The role of cystine-glutamate exchange in nicotine dependence in rats and humans. *Biological Psychiatry* 65(10):841-845.

Madayag, A., K.S. Kau, D. Lobner, et al. 2010. Drug-induced plasticity contributing to heightened relapse susceptibility: neurochemical changes and augmented reinstatement in high-intake rats. *Journal of Neuroscience* 30(1):210-217.

Mason, B. 2009. Effects of Gabapentin on cannabis withdrawal. Presented at Addiction Medicine State of the Art 2009.

Moore, S.C., L.M. Carter, and S.H.M. van Goozen. 2009. Confectionary consumption in childhood and adult violence. *British Journal of Psychiatry* 195:366-367; DOI: 10.1192/bjp.bp.108.061820.

Moussawi, K., A. Pacchioni, M. Moran, et al. 2009. N-Acetylcysteine reverses cocaine-induced metaplasticity. *Nature Neuroscience* 12(2):182-189.

Moussawi, K., W. Zhou, D.B. Carr, et al. 2009. N-acetylcysteine persistently prevents reinstatement of cacine seeking by countermanding cocaine induced synaptic potentiation in the nucleus accumbens. Presented at Neuroscience 2009, October, 19, 2009.

Raby, W.N., and S. Coomaraswamy. 2004. Gabapentin reduces cocaine use among addicts from a community clinic sample. *Journal of Clinical Psychiatry* 65(1):84-86.

Socker, S. 1999. Studies link stress and addiction. *NIDA Notes* 14(1).

Taylor, A.H., M.H. Ussher, and G. Faulkner. 2007. The acute effects of exercise on cigarette cravings, withdrawal symptoms, affect and smoking behaviour: A systematic review. *Addiction* 102(4):534-543.

Ussher, M.H., A. Taylor, and G. Faulkner. 2008. Exercise interventions for smoking cessation. *Cochrane Database of Systematic Reviews* (4):CD002295.

Uys, J.D., and R.T. LaLumiere. 2008. Glutamate: the new frontier in pharmacotherapy for cocaine addiction. *CNS & Neurological Disorders - Drug Targets* 7(5):482-491.

Van Rensburg, K.J., A. Taylor, and T. Hodgson. 2009. The effects of acute exercise on attentional bias towards smoking-related stimuli during temporary abstinence from smoking. *Addiction* 104(11):1910-1917.

Van Rensburg K.J., A. Taylor, T. Hodgson, et al. 2009. Acute exercise modulates cigarette cravings and brain activation in response to smoking-related images: An fMRI study. *Psychopharmacology* (Berl) 203(3):589-598.

Van Rensburg K.J., and A.H. Taylor. 2008. The effects of acute exercise on cognitive functioning and cigarette cravings during temporary abstinence from smoking. *Human Psychopharmacology* 23(3):193-199.

Wu, K.L., R. Chaikomin, S. Doran, et al. 2006. Artificially sweetened versus regular mixers increase gastric emptying and alcohol absorption. *The American Journal of Medicine* 119(9):802-804.

Zhou, W., and P.W. Kalivas. 2008. N-acetylcysteine reduces extinction responding and induces enduring reductions in cue- and heroin-induced drug-seeking. *Biological Psychiatry* 63(3):338-340.

CHAPTER 11

Ahmad, S.O., J.H. Park, J.D. Radel. 2008. Reduced numbers of dopamine neurons in the substantia nigra pars compacta and ventral tegmental area of rats fed an n-3 polyunsaturated fatty acid-deficient diet: a stereological study. *Neuroscience Letters* 438(3):30330-7.

Akhondzadeh, S., A. Basti, E. Moshiri, et al. 2007. Comparison of petal of Crocus sativus L. and fluoxetine in the treatment of depressed outpatients: a pilot double-blind randomized trial. *Progress in Neuro-Psychopharmacology and Biological Psychiatry* 31(2):439-442.

Akhondzadeh, S., N. Tahmacebi-Pour, A.A. Noorbala, et al. 2005. Crocus sativus L. in the treatment of mild to moderate depression: a double-blind, randomized and placebo-controlled trial. *Phytotherapy Research* 19(2):148-151.

Akhondzadeh, S., H. Fallah-Pour, K. Afkham, et al. 2004. Comparison of Crocus sativus L. and imipramine in the treatment of mild to moderate depression: a pilot double-blind randomized trial. *BMC Complementary and Alternative Medicine* 4:12.

Avena, N.M., P. Rada, and B.G. Hoebel. 2009. Sugar and fat bingeing have notable differences in addictive-like behavior. *Journal of Nutrition* 139(3):623-628.

Bello, N., et al. 2009. High-fat, high-sugar foods alter brain receptors. Presented at 2009 annual meeting of the Society for the Study of Ingestive Behavior.

Benoit, S.C, C.J. Kemp, C.F. Elias, et al. Palmitic acid mediates hypothalamic insulin resistance by altering PKC-θ subcellular localization in rodents. *The Journal of Clinical Investigation* 119(9):2577-2589.

Blaylock, R.L. *Excitotoxins: The Taste That Kills*. Santa Fe: Health Press, 1997.

Buydens-Branchey, L., M. Branchey, D.L. McMakin, et al. 2003. Polyunsaturated fatty acid status and relapse vulnerability in cocaine addicts. *Psychiatry Research* 120(1):29-35.

Estes, K.C., B.T. Rose, J.J. Speck, et al. 1997. Effects of omega 3 fatty acids on receptor tyrosine kinase and PLC activities in EMT6 cells. *Journal of Lipid Mediators and Cell Signaling* 17(2):81-96.

Fortuna, J. 2009. *Nutrition for the Focused Brain*. Cengage.

Fortuna, J. 1997 1st ed.; 1998 2nd ed. *Food, Brain Chemistry and Behavior*. Pearson.

Gaby, A. 1998. The role of hidden food allergy/intolerance in chronic disease. *Alternative Medicine Review* 3(2):90-100.

Gold, M.S., N.A. Graham, J.A. Cocores, et al. 2009. Food addiction? *Journal of Addiction Medicine* 3(1):42-45.

Ifland, J.R., H.G. Preuss, M.T. Marcus, et al. 2009. Refined food addiction: A classic substance use disorder. *Medical Hypotheses* 72(5):518-526.

Kennedy, D.O., Scholey, A.B. 2006. The psychopharmacology of European herbs with cognition-enhancing properties. *Current Pharmaceutical Design* 12(35):4613-4623.

Kessler, D. 2009. *The End of Overeating: Taking Control of the Insatiable American Appetite*. New York: Rodale Press.

Latagliata, E.C., E. Patrono, S. Puglisi-Allegra, et al. 2010. Food seeking in spite of harmful consequences is under prefrontal cortical noradrenergic control. *BMC Neuroscience* 11:15. DOI: 10.1186/1471-2202-11-15.

Masoumi, A., B. Goldenson, S. Ghirmai, et al. 2009. 25-dihydroxyvitamin D3 interacts with curcuminoids to stimulate amyloid-β clearance by macrophages of Alzheimer's disease patients. *Journal of Alzheimer's Disease* 17(3):703-717.

Moshiri, E., A.A. Basti, A.A.Noorbala, et al. 2006. Crocus sativus L. (petal) in the treatment of mild-to-moderate depression: a double-blind, randomized and placebo-controlled trial. *Phytomedicine* 13(9-10):607-611.

Mullarkey, B. How Safe Is Your Artificial Sweetener (account of John Cook), *Informed Consent Magazine* September/October 1994.

Peterson, D.W., R.C. George, F. Scaramozzino, et al. 2009. Cinnamon extract inhibits tau aggregation associated with Alzheimer's disease in vitro. *Journal of Alzheimer's Disease* 17(3):585-597.

Rapp, D. 1991. *Is This Your Child? Discovering and Treating Unrecognized Allergies in Children and Adults.* New York: Harper.

Von Deneen, K.M., M.S. Gold, and Y. Liu. 2009. Food addiction and cues in Prader-Willi Syndrome. *Journal of Addiction Medicine* 3(1):19–25.

Wurtman, R. 1988. *Dietary Phenylalanine and Brain Function: Proceedings of the First International Meeting on Dietary Phenylalanine and Brain Function.* Birkhauser.

CHAPTER 12

Brewer, J.A., R. Sinha, J.A. Chen, et al. 2009. Mindfulness training and stress reactivity in substance abuse: results from a randomized, controlled stage I pilot study. *Substance Abuse* 30(4):306-317.

Carroll, K.M., B.J.Rounsaville, C. Nich, et al. 1994. One year follow-up of psychotherapy and pharmacotherapy for cocaine dependence: Delayed emergence of psychotherapy effects. *Archives of General Psychiatry* 51(12):989-997.

Carroll, K.M., B.J. Rounsaville, and F.H. Gawin. 1991. A comparative trial of psychotherapies for ambulatory cocaine abusers: Relapse prevention and interpersonal psychotherapy. *American Journal of Drug and Alcohol Abuse* 17(3):229-247.

Hall, S.M., B.E. Havassy, and D.A. Wasserman. 1991 Effects of commitment to abstinence, positive moods, stress, and coping on relapse to cocaine use. *Journal of Consulting and Clinical Psychology* 59(4):526-532.

Higgins, S.T., D.D. Delaney, A.J. Budney, et al. 1991. A behavioral approach to achieving initial cocaine abstinence. *American Journal of Psychiatry* 148(9):1218-1224.

Kadden, R.M., N.L. Cooney, H. Getter, et al. 1989. Matching alcoholics to coping skills or interactional therapies: Post-treatment results. *Journal of Consulting and Clinical Psychology* 57(6):698-704.

Magill, M., and L.A. Ray. 2009. Cognitive-behavioral treatment with adult alcohol and illicit drug users: a meta-analysis of randomized controlled trials. *Journal of Studies on Alcohol and Drugs* 70(4):516-527.

Penberthy, J.K., N. Ait-Daoud, M. Vaughan, et al. 2010. Re-view of treatments for cocaine dependence. *Current Drug Abuse Reviews* published January 21, 2010. [Epub ahead of print]

Prochaska, J.O., C.C. DiClemente, and J.C. Norcross. 1992. In search of how people change: Applications to addictive behaviors. *American Psychologist* 47(9):1102-1114.

CHAPTER 13

Ahmed, S.H., and G.F. Koob. 1997. Cocaine- but not food-seeking behavior is reinstated by stress after extinction. *Psychopharmacology* 132(3):289-295.

Brewer, D.D., R.F. Catalano, K. Haggerty, et al. 1998. A meta-analysis of predictors of continued drug use during and after treatment for opiate addiction. *Addiction* 93(1):73-92.

Bowen, S., K. Witkiewitz, T.M. Dillworth, et al. 2006. Mindfulness meditation and substance use in an incarcerated population. *Psychology of Addictive Behaviors* 20(3):343-347.

Bowen, S., N. Chawla, S.E. Collins, et al. 2009. Mindfulness-based relapse prevention for substance use disorders: A pilot efficacy trial. *Substance Abuse* 30(4):295-305.

Chilcoat, H.D., and N. Breslau. 1998. Postraumatic stress disorder and drug disorders: Testing causal pathways. *Archives of General Psychiatry* 55(10):913-917.

Dawes, M.A., S.M. Antelman, M.M. Vanyukov, et al. 2000. Developmental sources of variation in liability to adolescent substance use disorders. *Drug and Alcohol Dependence* 61(1):3-14.

Deykin, E.Y., and S.L. Buka. 1997. Prevalence and risk factors for posttraumatic stress disorder among chemically dependent adolescents. *American Journal of Psychiatry* 154(6):752-757.

Erb, S., Y. Shaham, and J. Stewart. 1996. Stress reinstates cocaine-seeking behavior after prolonged extinction and a drug-free period. *Psychopharmacology* 128(4):408-412.

Jacobsen, L.K., S.M. Southwick, and T.R. Kosten. 2001. Substance use disorders in patients with posttraumatic stress disorder: A review of the literature. *American Journal of Psychiatry* 158(8):1184-1190.

Koob, G.F. 2010. The role of CRF and CRF-related peptides in the dark side of addiction. *Brain Research* 1314:3-14.

Koob, G.F. 2009. Brain stress systems in the amygdala and addiction. *Brain Research* 13;1293:61-75.

Koob, G., and M.J. Kreek. 2007. Stress, dysregulation of drug reward pathways, and the transition to drug dependence. *American Journal of Psychiatry* 164(8):1149-1159.

Kosten, T.R., B.J. Rounsaville, and H.D. Kleber. 1986. A 2.5 year follow-up of depressions, life crises, and treatment effects on abstinence among opioid addicts. *Archives of General Psychiatry* 43(8):733-739.

Lê, A.D., B. Quan, W. Juzytch, et al. 1998. Reinstatement of alcohol-seeking by priming injections of alcohol and exposure to stress in rats. *Psychopharmacology* 135(2):169-174.

Matheny, K.B., and K.E. Weatherman. 1998. Predictors of smoking cessation and maintenance. *Journal of Clinical Psychology* 54(2):223-235.

Piazza, P.V., and M. Le Moal. 1998.The role of stress in drug self-administration. *Trends in Pharmacological Sciences* 19(2):67-74.

Piazza, P.V., and M. Le Moal. 1996. Pathophysiological basis of vulnerability to drug abuse: role of an interaction between stress, glucocorticoids, and dopaminergic neurons. *Annual Review of Pharmacology and Toxicology* 36:359-378.

Piazza, P.V., J.M. Deminiere, M. Le Moal, et al. 1990. Stress- and pharmacologically-induced behavioral sensitization increases vulnerability to acquisition of amphetamine self-administration. *Brain Research* 514:22-26.

Shaham, Y., and J. Stewart. 1995 Stress reinstates heroin-seeking in drug-free animals: An effect mimicking heroin, not withdrawal. *Psychopharmacology* 119(3):334-341.

Sinha, R., D. Catapano, and S. O'Malley. 1999. Stress-induced craving and stress response in cocaine dependent individuals. *Psychopharmacology* 142(4):343-351.

Sinha, R., T. Fuse, L.R. Aubin, et al. 2000. Psychological stress, drug-related cues, and cocaine craving. *Psychopharmacology* 152(2):140-148.

Stewart, J. 2000. Pathways to relapse: The neurobiology of drug- and stress-induced relapse to drug-taking. *Journal of Psychiatry & Neuroscience* 25(2):125-136.

CHAPTER 14

Goldsmith, R.J., and J. Knapp. 1993. Towards a broader view of recovery. *Journal of Substance Abuse Treatment* 10(2):107-111.

McIlvain, H.E., J.K. Bobo, A. Leed-Kelly, et al. 1998. Practical steps to smoking cessation for recovering alcoholics. *American Family Physician* April 15, 1998.

Reich, M.S., M.S. Dietrich, A.J. Finlayson, et al. 2008. Coffee and cigarette consumption and perceived effects in recovering alcoholics participating in Alcoholics Anonymous in Nashville, Tennessee, USA. *Alcohol, Clinical and Experimental Research* 32(10):1799-1806.

Sinha, R., M. Talih, R. Malison, et al. 2003. Hypothalamic-pituitary-adrenal axis and sympatho-adreno-medullary responses during stress-induced and drug cue-induced cocaine craving states. *Psychopharmacology* (Berl). 170(1):62-72.

CHAPTER 15

Fals-Stewart, W., T.J. O'Farrell, and G.R. Birchler. 2004. Behavioral couples therapy for substance abuse: rationale, methods, and findings. *Science & Practice Perspectives* 2(2):30-41.

O'Farrell, T.J., M. Murphy, J. Alter, et al. 2010. Behavioral family counseling for substance abuse: a treatment development pilot study. *Addictive Behaviors* 35(1):1-6.

Petry, N.M., and L. Weiss. 2009. Social support is associated with gambling treatment outcomes in pathological gamblers. *American Journal on Addictions* 18(5):402-408.

Powers, M.B., E. Vedel, P.M. Emmelkamp. 2008. Behavioral couples therapy (BCT) for alcohol and drug use disorders: a meta-analysis. *Clinical Psychology Review* 28(6):952-962.

APPENDIX B

Atack, J.R. 2003. Anxioselective compounds acting at the GABA (A) receptor benzodiazepine binding site. *Current Drug Targets. CNS and Neurological Disorders* 2(4):213-232.

Aydin, K., S. Kircan, S. Sarwar, et al. 2009. Smaller gray matter volumes in frontal and parietal cortices of solvent abusers correlate with cognitive deficits. *AJNR American Journal of Neuroradiology* 30(10):1922-1928.

Barrett, S.P., C. Darredeau, L.E. Bordy, et al. 2005. Characteristics of methylphenidate misuse in a university student sample. *Canadian Journal of Psychiatry* 50:457–461.

Boyd, C.J., S.E. McCabe, J.A. Cranford, et al. 2007. Prescription drug abuse and diversion among adolescents in a southeast Michigan school district. *Archives of Pediatric and Adolescent Medicine* 161:276–281.

Briken, P., and R. Basdekis-Jozsa. 2010. Sexual addiction? When sexual behavior gets out of control. *Bundesgesundheitsblatt Gesundheitsforschung Gesundheitsschutz* March 4, 2100 [E-pub ahead of print].

Clark, L., A.J. Lawrence, F. Astley-Jones, et al. 2009. Gambling near-misses enhance motivation to gamble and recruit win-related brain circuitry. *Neuron* 61(3):481-490.

Filley, C.M., W. Halliday, and B.K. Kleinschmidt-DeMasters. 2004. The effects of toluene on the central nervous system. *Journal of Neuropathology and Experimental Neurology* 2004 Jan;63(1):1-12.

Gelderloos, P., K.G. Walton, D.W. Orme-Johnson, et al. 1991. Effectiveness of the Transcendental Meditation program in preventing and treating substance misuse: A review. *International Journal of Addictions* 26(3):293-325.

Gerada, C., and M. Ashworth. 1997. ABC of mental health. Addiction and dependence—I: Illicit drugs. *BMJ* 315(7107):297-300.

Gerasimov, M.R., R.A. Ferrieri, W.K. Schiffer, et al. 2002. Study of brain uptake and biodistribution of [11C]toluene in non-human primates and mice. *Life Sciences* 70(23):2811-2828.

Guay, D.R. 2009. Drug treatment of paraphilic and nonparaphilic sexual disorders. *Clinical Therapeutics* 31(1):1-31.

Herrera, D.G., A.G. Yague, S. Johnsen–Soriano, et al. 2003. Selective impairment of hippocampal neurogenesis by chronic alcoholism: Protective effects of an antioxidant. Proceedings of the National Academy of Science of the U.S.A. 100(13):7919–7924, 2003.

Hommer, D.W. Male and female sensitivity to alcohol–induced brain damage. Alcohol Research & Health 27(2):181–185, 2003.

Jacobson, R. 1986. The contributions of sex and drinking history to the CT brain scan changes in alcoholics. Psychological Medicine 16:547–559.

Jupp, B., and A.J. Lawrence. 2010. New horizons for therapeutics in drug and alcohol abuse. *Pharmacology and Therapeutics* 125(1):138-68.

Little, K.Y., D. M. Krolewski, L. Zhang, et al. 2003. Loss of striatal vesicular monoamine transporter protein (VMAT2) in human cocaine users. *American Journal of Psychiatry* 160:47-55.

Lowery, E.G., and T.E. Thiele. 2010. Pre-clinical evidence that corticotropin-releasing factor (CRF) receptor antagonists are promising targets for pharmacological treatment of alcoholism. *CNS & Neurological Disorders Drug Targets* 9(1):77-86.

Lurie, M.D., and P.R. Lee. 1991. Fifteen solutions to the problems of prescription drug abuse. *Journal of Psychoactive Drugs* 23(4):349-357.

Mann, K., A. Batra, A. Gunther, and G. Schroth. 1992. Do women develop alcoholic brain damage more readily than men? *Alcoholism: Clinical and Experimental Research* 16(6):1052–1056.

Moreno, I., J. Saiz-Ruiz, and J.J. Lopez-Ibor. 2004. Serotonin and gambling dependence. *Human Psychopharmacology: Clinical and Experimental* 6(S1):S9-S12. DOI: 10.1002/hup.470060 503.

National Council on Problem Gambling. http://www.ncpgambling.org/i4a/pages/Index.cfm?pageID=3315#widespread

National Health Interview Survey (NHIS). 2008, National Center for Health Statistics NIDA (National Institute on Drug Abuse),

U.S. Department of Health and Human Services/National Institutes of Health. 2007. *Drugs, Brains, and Behavior: The Science of Addiciton.* NIH Publication #07-5605.

Nixon, K., and F.T. Crews. 2002. Binge ethanol exposure decreases neurogenesis in adult rat hippocampus. Journal of Neurochemistry 83(5):1087–1093.

Nixon, S., R. Tivis, and O. Parsons. 1995. Behavioral dysfunction and cognitive efficiency in male and female alcoholics. Alcoholism: Clinical and Experimental Research 19(3):577–558.

NSDUH. 2006. Drug and alcohol use: 2006 National Survey on Drug Use and Health, Office of Applied Studies. NSDUH Series H-32, DHHS Publication No. SMA 07-4293.

O'Brien, C.P. 2005. Benzodiazepine use, abuse, and dependence. *Journal of Clinical Psychiatry* 66(Suppl 2):28-33.

Petry, N.M., and L. Weiss. 2009. Social support is associated with gambling treatment outcomes in pathological gamblers. *American Journal on Addictions* 18(5):402-408.

Pettinati, H.M., D.W. Oslin, K.M. Kampman, et al. 2010. A double-blind, placebo-controlled trial combining sertraline and naltrexone for treating co-occurring depression and alcohol dependence. *American Journal of Psychiatry* published online March 15, 2010. DOI: 10.1176/appi.ajp.2009.08060852.

Raji, C.A., A.J. Ho, N.N. Parikshak, et al. 2009. Brain structure and obesity. *Human Brain Mapping* 31(3):353-364. DOI: 10.1002/hbm.20870.

Ries, R., D. Fiellin, S. Miller, et al. 2009. *Principles of Addiction Medicine, 4th Edition.* Lippincott, Williams & Wilkins.

SAMHSA. 2010. New national study reveals 12 year olds more likely to use potentially deadly inhalants than cigarettes or marijuana. March 11, 2010.

Seo, H.S., M. Yang, M.S. Song, et al. 2010. Toluene inhibits hippocampal neurogenesis in adult mice. *Pharmacology, Biochemistry and Behavior* 94(4):588-594.

Subrahmanyam, S., M. Satyanarayana, and K.R. Rajeswari. 1986. Alcoholism: Newer methods of management. *Indian Journal of Physiology and Pharmacology* 30(1):43-54.

U.S. Department of Health & Human Services. 2004. Alcohol's damaging effects on the brain. *Alcohol Alert* 63.

Wesson, D.R., and D.E. Smith. 1990. Prescription drug abuse: Patient, physician, and cultural responsibilities. *Addiction Medicine* 152:613-616.

White, B.P., K.A. Becker-Blease, and K. Grace-Bishop. 2006. Stimulant medication use, misuse, and abuse in an undergraduate and graduate student sample. *Journal of American College Health* 54:261–268.

Williams, S.H. 2005. Medications for treating alcohol dependence. *American Family Physician* 72:1775-1780.

APPENDIX C

Jarrell, N. 2009. A healing triangle. *Addiction Professional* 7(1): 15-20.

ORGANIZATIONS

Alliance for Addiction Solutions
www.allianceforaddictionsolutions.org

This is a nonprofit organization of physicians, counselors, acupuncturists and other health professionals using nutritional supplements, nourishing foods, and other mind-body integration methods to address the core biological needs of people in addiction and recovery.

Newport Academy
www.newport-academy.com
866.382.6651

Newport Academy is a gender-specific, comprehensive, residential treatment program for teens suffering from substance abuse and co-occurring disorders. Newport Academy is dedicated to providing integrated treatment programs in a caring and compassionate environment by which teens and their families may recover from the destructive effects of addictive disease and related behavioral health issues. David E. Smith, MD, is the chair of addiction medicine at Newport Academy.

NIDA
www.drugabuse.gov

NIDA looks at the science behind drug abuse and addiction. NIDA offers the latest cutting-edge findings and research in a variety of educational publications and formats geared to parents, children, adolescents, young adults, and teachers.

Partnership for a Drug-Free America
www.drugfree.org

The Partnership for a Drug-Free America is a nonprofit organization that unites parents, renowned scientists and communications professionals to help families raise healthy children. Best known for its research-based national public education programs, the Partnership motivates and equips parents to prevent their children from using drugs and alcohol, and to find help and treatment for family and friends in trouble.

Substance Abuse & Mental Health Services Association (SAMHSA)
www.samhsa.gov

http://findtreatment.samhsa.gov (substance abuse treatment facility locator)
24-hour helpline: 800-662-HELP (800-662-4357)

The Substance Abuse and Mental Health Services Administration (SAMHSA) offers a variety of assistance for people with addictions. There is a substance abuse treatment facility locator to help you find help in your area and a 24-hour helpline you can call when you are in need.

ACKNOWLEDGMENTS

I am grateful to the many people who have been instrumental in making this book a reality, especially all of the patients and professionals who have taught me so much about how the brain relates to addictions. I am especially grateful to our writing partner Frances Sharpe who was invaluable in the collaboration process between David and myself. She is truly a treasure. I am also grateful to David Smith, his wife Millicent and son Christopher, whom I have loved for a long time.

Our staff at Amen Clinics, Inc., as always, provided tremendous help and support during this process, especially my personal assistant Catherine Hanlon, Jackie Frattali, Corey Liebig, and our research director, Dr. Kristen Willeumier.

I am also grateful to Dr. Robert Johnson, Medical Director of Sierra Tucson, who embraced brain SPECT imaging technology and has used it to help his patients at Sierra Tucson! In addition, I am grateful that Dr. Jeff Fortuna of California State University Fullerton generously shared his knowledge of nutrition and addiction and significantly enhance our program. Christopher Buxton-Smith, the executive chef at Newport Academy during this writing project, was also very helpful in recording the CDs of the program and sharing his wisdom on nutrition and addiction.

I am also sincerely grateful to my literary agent Faith Hamlin, who besides being one of my best friends is a thoughtful, protective, creative mentor, along with the whole team at Sanford J. Greenburger Associates for their longstanding love, support, and guidance.

And, to Tana—my wife, my joy, and my best friend—who patiently listened to me for hours on end and gave many thoughtful suggestions on the book. I love all of you. — Daniel

•••••

I couldn't have contributed to this volume without the foundation laid during the past forty-some years of thousands of people—from the physicians at the University of California San Francisco and the San Francisco Medical Society who supported my vision of making health care a right, not a privilege, and opening the Haight Ashbury Free Medical Clinic; to the staff, volunteers, and patients of the clinic who provided such a rich resource for the evolution of my philosophy of addictive disease. My many colleagues in bringing Addiction Medicine to recognition as a mainstream medical specialty must also be acknowledged.

I am grateful to Don Wesson, MD, for his many years of sharing his research and writing expertise. I thank Rick Seymour for his long-standing roles as my support in recovery and co-author extraordinaire. Steve Heilig and Scott Sowle have provided invaluable perception and counsel. Terry Chambers, Jeffrey H. Novey, and Leif Zerkin, as current and past editors of the *Journal of Psychoactive Drugs,* have supplied significant information about substances falling outside the mainstream literature.

Dr. Jeffrey Fortuna and Christopher Buxton-Smith offered new insights into the role of food in addiction. Suzanne C. Smith; Bob Student; Glenn "Raz" Raswyck, EMT; and Leigh Davidson have lent their considerable organizational, research, and technical skills. Frances Sharpe has played an essential role in making this book a reality.

Finally, I thank my wife, Millicent Buxton-Smith, for her patience with my many projects and dreams. Working side by side with me to educate health professionals regarding diagnostic issues and the evaluation and treatment of impaired clinicians, she has shared her extensive expertise in the recovery field to help addicts break the bonds of their dependency. — David

ABOUT THE AUTHORS

Daniel G. Amen, MD

Daniel G. Amen, MD, is a physician, child and adult psychiatrist, brain imaging specialist, and *New York Times* bestselling author. He is the writer, producer, and host of four highly successful public television programs, raising more than $20 million for public television. He is a Distinguished Fellow of the American Psychiatric Association and the CEO and medical director of Amen Clinics in Newport Beach and Fairfield, California; Tacoma, Washington; and Reston, Virginia.

Amen Clinics is the world leader in applying brain imaging science to everyday clinical practice and has the world's largest database of functional scans related to behavior, now totaling more than 57,000.

Dr. Amen is the author of 35 professional scientific articles and 24 books, including the *New York Times* bestsellers, *Change Your Brain, Change Your Body; Change Your Brain, Change Your Life;* and *Magnificent Mind At Any Age.* He is also the author of *Healing ADD, Healing the Hardware of the Soul, Making a Good Brain Great, The Brain In Love*, and the co-author of *Healing Anxiety And Depression* and *Preventing Alzheimer's.*

Dr. Amen has appeared on The Dr. Oz Show, the Dr. Phil show, The Rachael Ray Show, the Today Show, Good Morning America, The View, Larry King, The Early Show, CNN, HBO, Discovery Channel, and many other national television and radio programs. His national public television shows include Change Your Brain, Change Your Life; Magnificent Mind At Any Age; The Brain In Love; and Change Your Brain, Change Your Body.

A small sample of the organizations Dr. Amen has spoken for include the National Security Agency (NSA); the National Science

Foundation (NSF); Harvard's Learning and the Brain Conference; The Million Dollar Roundtable; Retired NFL Players Summit; and the Supreme Courts of Delaware, Ohio, and Wyoming.

Dr. Amen has been featured in *Newsweek*, *Parade Magazine*, the *New York Times Magazine*, *Men's Health,* and *Cosmopolitan.*

Dr. Amen is married, the father of four children, grandfather to Elias, and an avid table tennis player.

David E. Smith, MD

David E. Smith, MD, has been at the forefront of Addiction Medicine since 1967. After seeing first hand the ravages of unchecked drug use during and especially following the Summer of Love, he has worked tirelessly to develop new treatment approaches to addictive disease and has advocated successfully for recognition of addiction as a brain disease. He is a Diplomate of the American Board of Addiction Medicine, a Fellow of the American Society of Addiction Medicine, and a Fellow of the American Academy of Clinical Toxicology. Dr. Smith is the Chair of Addiction Medicine at Newport Academy and Medical Director of Center Point. He is the Founder and former Medical Director of the Haight Ashbury Free Medical Clinic.

Dr. Smith has authored and co-authored over 350 professional articles and over two dozen books, including *It's So Good, Don't Even Try It Once: Heroin in Perspective*; *The Physician's Guide to Psychoactive Drugs; Drugfree: A Unique, Positive Approach to Staying Off Alcohol and Other Drugs*; and *Clinician's Guide to Substance Abuse.*

Dr. Smith has also served as President of the American Society of Addiction Medicine and the California Society of Addiction Medicine. He has held appointments with the University of California, San Francisco; the State of California Alcohol and

Drug Programs; National Institutes of Drug Abuse; and many other institutions and organizations.

Among the many organizations for which Dr. Smith has recently presented lectures are the American Psychiatric Association, the Utah District Court Judges Conference and Criminal Defense Lawyers, and the Conference on Behavioral Health & Addictive Disorders. He is also on the faculty of the ASAM Medical Review Officer Training courses.

Dr. Smith is married; the father of four children; grandfather to Lauren, Ashton, and Alexander; and a passionate basketball player (Platinum League), skier, scuba diver, and golfer.

Amen Clinics, Inc.

Amen Clinics, Inc. (ACI) was established in 1989 by Daniel G. Amen, MD. They specialize in innovative diagnosis and treatment planning for a wide variety of behavioral, learning, emotional and cognitive, and weight problems for children, teenagers, and adults. ACI has an international reputation for evaluating brain-behavior problems, such as attention deficit disorder (ADD), depression, anxiety, school failure, brain trauma, obsessive-compulsive disorders, aggressiveness, marital conflict, cognitive decline, brain toxicity from drugs or alcohol, and obesity. Brain SPECT imaging is performed in the Clinics. ACI has the world's largest database of brain scans for behavioral problems.

ACI welcome referrals from physicians, psychologists, social workers, marriage and family therapists, drug and alcohol counselors, and individual clients.

Amen Clinics, Inc., Newport Beach
4019 Westerly Place, Suite 100
Newport Beach, CA 92660
Toll-free: (888) 564-2700

Amen Clinics, Inc., Fairfield
350 Chadbourne Road
Fairfield, CA 94534
Toll-free: (888) 564-2700

Amen Clinics, Inc., Northwest
3315 South 23rd Street, Suite 102
Tacoma, WA 98405
Toll-free: (888) 564-2700

Amen Clinics, Inc., DC
1875 Campus Commons Drive, Suite 101
Reston, VA 20191
Toll-free: (888) 564-2700

Amenclinic.com

Amenclinic.com is an educational interactive brain website geared toward mental health and medical professionals, educators, students, and the general public. It contains a wealth of information to help you learn about our clinics and the brain. The site contains over 300 color brain SPECT images, thousands of scientific abstracts on brain SPECT imaging for psychiatry, a brain puzzle, and much, much more.

View over 300 astonishing color 3-D brain SPECT images on:
Aggression
Attention Deficit Disorder, including the six subtypes
Dementia and cognitive decline
Drug Abuse
PMS
Anxiety Disorders
Brain Trauma
Depression
Obsessive-Compulsive Disorder
Stroke
Seizures